DON'T FEEL LIKE A PRICK?
By Lynn Santer

A WORD ON THE COVER GRAPHIC

I have been asked why I chose a needle in the arm as opposed to the most common site for insulin injections (the subcutaneous fat of the stomach) or the most common site for the glucose test by lancet (the finger) on the cover. The reason is that one of the objectives of this title is to encourage people to get a blood test (the needle in the *arm*) to find out if they are one of the undiagnosed Type Two diabetics or pre-diabetics walking around with a time bomb inside waiting to explode. So... now you know.

**Cover design and cartoons
by Brett Sherwell
www.sherwellgraphics.com.au**

Photography (on Tanna) by Andrew Jacob

**Edited by Karen O'Brien
kareno247@gmail.com**

"If you don't have diabetes, you probably know someone who does, even if they don't know it yet. Everyone should read this book!"

- Karen O'Brien

Diabetes doesn't pounce on a person out of the blue. Before the diagnosis, a person may linger on the fringes of the condition with high blood sugar but not yet over that line that is clearly diabetes — for years. The U.S. Centers for Disease Control and Prevention released figures in January 2012 showing that the number of American adults with pre-diabetes had jumped from 57 million in 2008 to 79 million in 2010. During the same period, the number with full-on diabetes grew from 23.6 million to 26 million, the vast majority of which are Type 2 cases.

ABOUT THE AUTHOR

Lynn Santer is a novelist, biographer, ghost writer, celebrity manager, screenwriter, film producer, founder of The Magical Scarecrows "Let's Make Magic" programs for disabled and disadvantaged children, a wildlife conservation crusader, founder of the "Passion for Peace" program comprised of Saddam Hussein's former personal pilot, an ultra orthodox Israeli Rabbi and a spokesperson from World Vision, a nominee for the Pride of Australia medal… and she is also a diabetic.

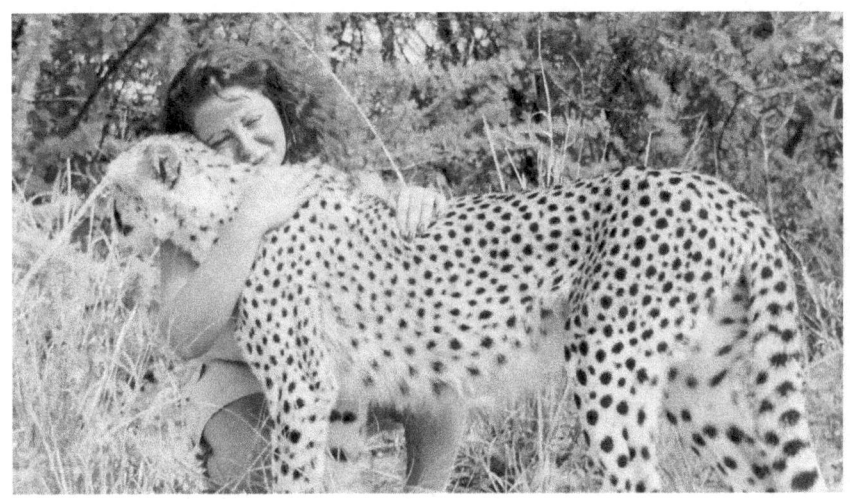

A PERCENTAGE OF ALL PROCEEDS FROM THIS BOOK WILL BE DONATED TO DIABETES RESEARCH

In Australia alone it is estimated there are currently 680,000 undiagnosed Type Two diabetics and *two (2) million* pre-diabetics. In the US the number of pre-diabetics is almost *eighty (80) million* people and in Britain it is seven million people. People are not being tested because diabetes frequently shows no symptoms yet according to the Bureau of Statistics diabetes is in the *top ten causes of death*.

According to the National Diabetes Statistics (US Government) more than half of the deaths caused by diabetes do not list diabetes as the cause of death – rather they list the condition brought on my diabetes (such as heart attack or stroke) as the cause of death. They also state the risk of death among people with diabetes is *twice* that of a person the same age without diabetes.
http://diabetes.niddk.nih.gov/dm/pubs/statistics/#Deaths

Only having an *annual* blood test will ensure you keep on top of what is happening in your body. Currently there is *no cure* for diabetes but it *can* be controlled. To avoid complications that can set in prior to diagnosis simply have an annual test.

Annual blood tests are **FREE**
(in Australia)

The life you save by taking or passing on the advice in this book could be yours… or it could be the life of someone you love.

CONTENTS

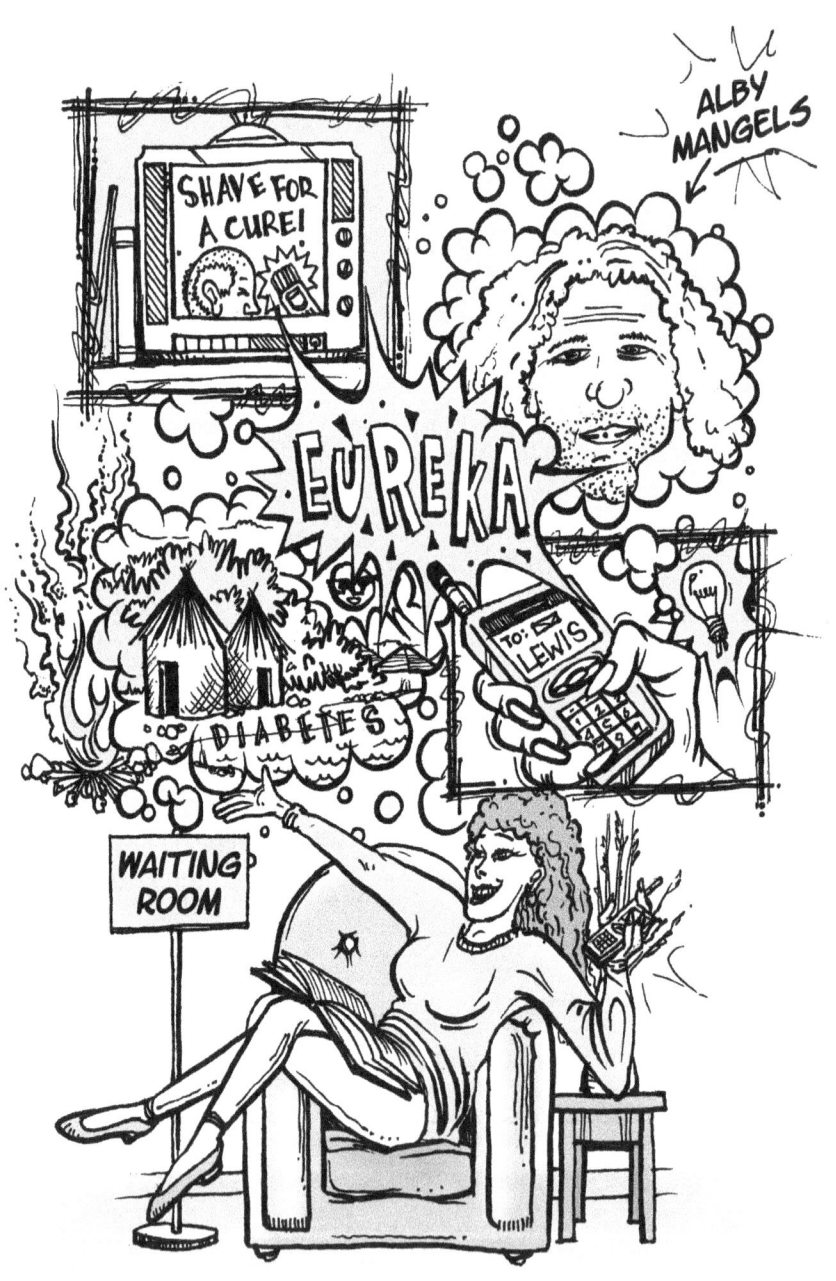

INTRODUCTION

You might be wondering how I came up with the title for this book. Well… I'll tell you. I was sitting in my gynaecologist's waiting room, watching TV. I had already begun work on a co-production with Alby Mangels for a film we are developing in collaboration with Lewis Kaplan, the CEO of Diabetes Australia, about (curiously enough) diabetes. (I'll talk more about the film later.) A commercial flashed on TV about the Leukaemia Foundation's "Shave for a Cure" day. I found my creative juices following a thought sequence and maybe, just maybe, there might have been some vague association occurring in the back of my mind apropos of where I was. Suddenly I almost yelled "Eureka!" as the idea came to me. I was so pleased with my brain spark I immediately sent Lewis a text message. He was responding just as I was called for my appointment. Lewis not only thoroughly approved but was highly amused by my idea (albeit he didn't have a clue where I was or how I came up with this brain spark). I was giggling at Lewis' response as I sat down opposite my gyno. You can imagine this is not particularly a reaction he is used to!

Feeling the need to explain myself, or at least explain why I was giggling at a rather inappropriate time, I turned my phone around and showed my gyno the sequence of text messages. He couldn't wipe the grin off his face, which given the benefit of hindsight might not have been entirely the most intelligent thing I could have done as I'd probably rather his hands weren't trembling with laughter! For those of you who don't know who Alby Mangels is and why this is even funnier when you do know I will explain later on in this book. It took a bit of convincing Alby to accept the title, as his face was to be associated with it, but with the reaction we received consistently from that moment on it has been hard to imagine it could ever have been called anything else.

IT DOESN'T HAVE TO BE DIFFICULT

I know when you are first diagnosed there is an information explosion and much of the information is dry, technical and frankly overwhelming. On top of that the statistics can be terrifying. However, you don't have to be terrified and you don't have to be overwhelmed. What you do have to be is aware and vigilant. It really isn't that hard to get things right and the number of famous people who have lived long and happy lives with diabetes prove this point. Just take a look at the list:

George Lucas – creator of "Star Wars"
Elizabeth Taylor
Sharon Stone
Peter O'Toole
Cathy Freeman – Olympic Gold Medallist (running)
Johnny Cash
Mikhail Gorbachev
Jack Benny
Halle Berry
HG Wells
Thomas Edison
James Cagney
Jerry Lewis
Mary Tyler Moore
Spencer Tracy
Mae West
Jane Wyman
Carol Channing
Sugar Ray Robinson – World Champion Boxer
Arthur Ashe – Wimbledon Tennis Champion
Billie Jean King – Wimbledon Tennis Champion
Sir Steve Redgrave – 5 time Olympic gold medallist (rowing)
Gary Hall – Olympic gold medallist (swimming)
Doug Burns – Mr Universe
And the list goes on… and on…

My last birthday party was catered. The originally suggested canapé menu looked like this:

- Mini profiteroles with smoked ham and Swiss cheese
- Creamed corn and asparagus in mini cobs
- Chicken sates with peanut dipping sauce
- Steamed prawn dumplings with sweet chilli and coriander dipping sauce
- Spinach and feta filo triangles
- Mini hash browns topped with smoked salmon and sour cream
- Soy and garlic grilled beef fillet
- Chicken and green onion meatballs with honey and lemon pepper glaze
- Birthday cake

To change this to diabetic friendly all I had to do was:

- ✓ Exchange Swiss cheese for lowest fat Swiss cheese
- ✓ Ensure there was no sugar in the peanut dipping sauce
- ✓ Change the sweet chilli and coriander dipping sauce to a non-sweet dipping sauce
- ✓ Use low fat sour cream for the smoked salmon
- ✓ Change the glaze on the chicken and green onion meatballs to one without honey
- ✓ Ditch the birthday cake and serve diabetic chocolate in squares with strawberries surrounding it and sparklers shooting out the sides… and it looked amazing!

How easy was that? (And being me I had to insist all the meat was free range too.)

Even in this simple book there is a lot of information and some frightening truths but I've tried to make it easy, fun and realistic for real people living real lives in the real world. So let us embark together on this journey…

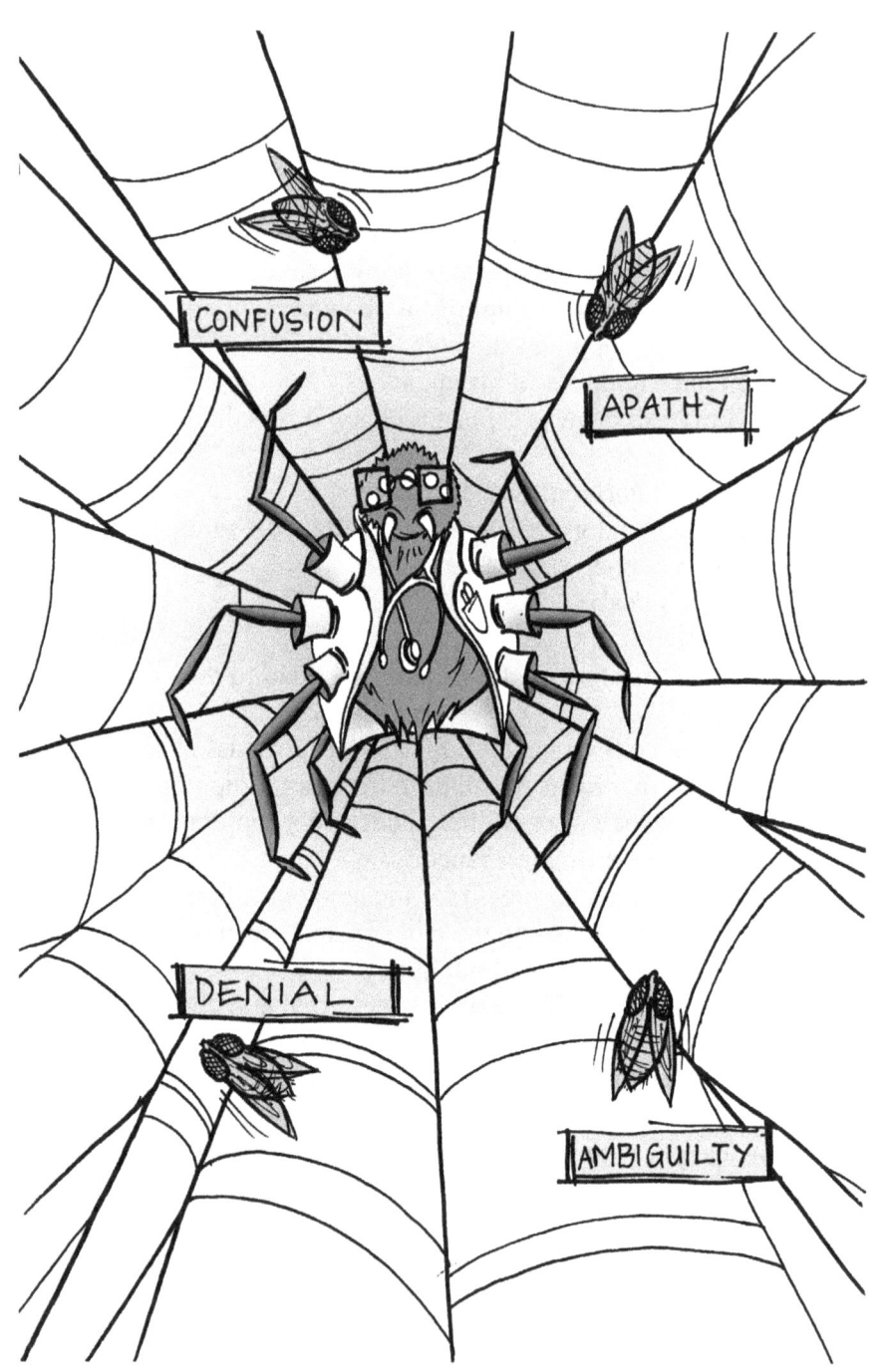

QUALIFYING NOTE

I would like to preface *everything* I am going to say in the early chapters of this book about thin, young, active people being diagnosed with Type Two diabetes by saying please read the chapter on *LATENT AUTOIMMUNE DIABETES OF ADULTS (LADA)* and consider whether this might apply to you – or indeed the other case studies that I refer to.

Diabetes is a very complex condition. There is no simple "one size fits all" to effectively managing it. My aim in this book is to take you through some of the possible methods that might help you, explain some of the techniques that have helped me, give you a few tips along the way, hopefully give you a giggle here and there and generally demystify the spider's web of confusion, ambiguity, apathy and denial that exists in the general populous.

This is one condition that definitely should *not* be "sugar-coated" – every pun intended.

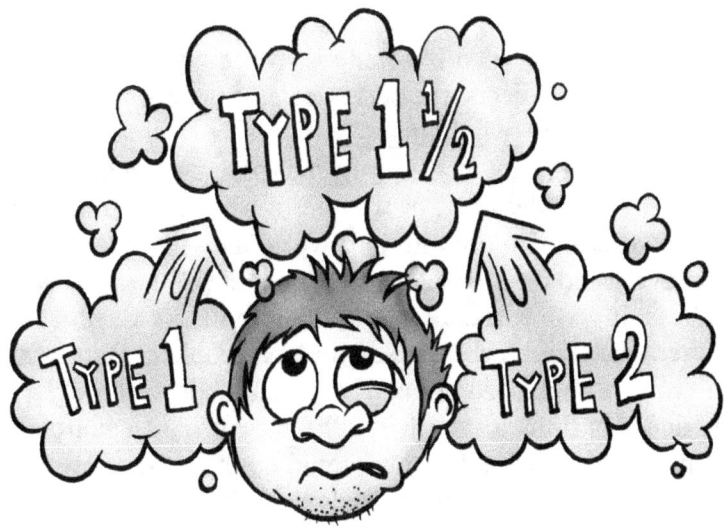

INCH BY INCH ANYTHING'S A CINCH

We all know that if we did everything our doctor, diabetic educator, dietitian, dentist, podiatrist, beautician, hairdresser, etc told us to do before we went out in the morning it would probably be time to go back to bed. We all have busy lives and none of us are perfect – I'm certainly not! But does that mean we do nothing? Does that mean we bury our heads in the sand because the pain and suffering that can come with diabetes isn't manifesting itself as a clear and present danger we are forced to address in the "now"? Okay, life might become as boring as proverbial doggie doo if we religiously did everything we are told, but just because we can't or won't take every piece of advice we're given, doesn't mean we can't start taking one piece of advice and build up momentum from there.

Every drop makes up the ocean. The journey of a thousand miles starts with the first step. Every single piece of advice you do take is going to help you live the life you want to live.

Many years ago, when I became involved with various philanthropic projects, the sheer scale of the problems at hand seemed overwhelming. Whether it be trying to save endangered big cats in Africa from brutal, unethical and illegal forms of hunting, or whether it be bringing medical aid to suffering children in third world nations, it seemed whatever I did or gave it was never enough – the need was endless. It was profoundly depressing to think that no matter what I did there would still be a problem. But does that mean I should do nothing? Certainly not! If through my deeds or donations only one life is saved, safeguarded or improved, it's one life that would not have been saved, safeguarded or improved if I'd done nothing.

A very wise man, by the name of Ralph Waldo Emerson, a nineteenth century philosopher and poet, said:

"If one life has breathed easier because you have lived – this is to have succeeded."

Today we are going to talk about the life which breathes easier because you have lived being... YOU.

The key things are:

- Time Management (to be physically active),
- Discipline (to eat only the right things), and
- Motivation (what's the one thing that means more to you than anything?)

To be physically active you might need to get into the habit of getting up half an hour earlier, or going to bed half an hour later in order to walk or swim or do something that gets your circulation going for 30 minutes a day. It really isn't that hard and if you're a multi-tasker you can still do text messages while you're walking, have someone sit on the side of the pool to take notes for you while you're having ideas during your swim, or you could just relax and enjoy the great outdoors discovering there are sights and sounds and smells you've never noticed before! But, manage your time to ensure you can do something physically active for 30 minutes every day.

Discipline is a matter of training your mind. If you like, it's a form of self-hypnosis. Think of the thing that frightens you the most – what if you were physically incapable of taking the kids to school, or playing your favourite musical instrument, or let's get down to one of the best primal motivators for all (most) of us – what if you were unable to have sex anymore? Oh yes, that's right, one of the many possible complications of diabetes you rarely hear about is decreased libido and impotence – and who wants that? If every time you're tempted to have that piece of chocolate you shouldn't have, or that delicious looking sauce you know is loaded with sugar and/or cholesterol, if every time you were about to indulge thinking, "It's only once – what harm can it do?" instead of thinking that, train your brain to trigger with the thought, "If I eat that I'm bringing the day forward when I won't be able to……." whatever it is that works for you. You will astonish yourself at how you are no longer even tempted to eat the foods you shouldn't eat. Don't do it because your doctor says so. Who cares what your doctor thinks? Do it because it matters… **to you**. You will soon discover that not only are you not so much as tempted to eat the wrong foods any more, you will notice when everyone around you is drinking a sugary drink, eating fatty foods, or otherwise screwing up their future, and you'll find yourself wanting to yell, "Stop it! Don't you realise what you're doing to yourself?"

The best motivation of all comes in the form of whatever it is that tugs at your heart strings the most. Everyone has something or someone who does that. I will share with you my very personal motivation just to get you thinking about what it might be that works for you – perhaps vaguely along the same lines or perhaps for you it's something completely different. When my father lay dying of complications from diabetes in hospital it wasn't pretty. He had been the centre of my world, my role model, my hero, a man of intense dignity, integrity, honesty, courage, strength and success. There was no one I admired or respected (or dare I say was even intimidated by) more. At one point during those final days I stumbled outside his hospital room, fell to my knees, bowed my head and wept into my hands like a baby at his pain. Now I have two nephews who believe that Auntie Lynn can in fact actually walk on water. "Who's the best aunt in the whole world?" I have been asking them almost since birth. In unison the reply is always a robust, "Auntie Lynn!" Our bond is so tight it is something very, very special indeed. Of course sooner or later we all have to die, but there's a time and there's a way and I can't bear the thought that some time in the future my nephews will be by my hospital bed and stumbling outside the room, falling to their knees and weeping into their hands at their aunt's fate. If you don't care about you – how much do you care about the people who care about you?

There are, I believe, many among us who would be prepared to lay down our own lives for something we feel passionately about (a country, a cause, a great leader… the right to wear fur-lined underwear in the Antarctic – whatever) but how many of us would lay down the life of someone we loved for that thing we feel passionate about? Or look at it another way – I would refuse an organ transplant from an animal, even if it was to save my life, because that animal wasn't being given the choice – that just happens to be my belief. But would I refuse that animal organ transplant if it was going to save the life of one of my nephews? Absolutely not! The point is that sometimes it is easier to ignore your own wellbeing without realising that no person is an island. If your thread of life is pulled out from the tapestry of people in your world, something else will unravel. If doing it for you isn't what's going to motivate you – then do it for that special person in your life whose world might stop turning if you weren't in it – or if you became incapacitated – or if you were suffering unendurable pain. Think about that!

Hum – I did promise there would be some fun and laughs in this book, didn't I? Okay, let's get off the soap box for a minute and look at something else…

Just in case you think you're the only one out there who isn't taking your condition as seriously as you should, get a load of this. My gyno (aforementioned in the introduction) is refusing to have a regular test for diabetes because he doesn't want to know about it. My G.P. confessed to me he hasn't had his latest cholesterol check because he didn't want to know the result. My optician's assistant told me he had diabetes once but cured it in three months and so now he's back on a family-sized bar of chocolate a day! That's our esteemed medical professionals who are supposed to lead by example! Talk about the proverbial tailor without the trousers! You've heard the old saying, haven't you, "What's the difference between God and a doctor? God doesn't think he's a doctor!" So come on people, let *us* show *them* how to be responsible and do it right – how would that be for a turn up for the books, hey?

FYI – currently diabetes can *not* be cured. I will talk more about that later, but good management and control are *not* a cure – it is inaccurate and irresponsible to think or say otherwise.

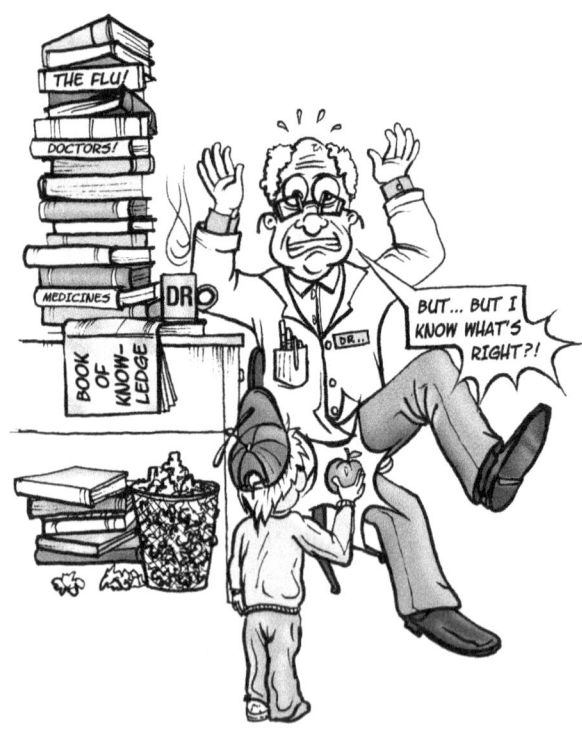

IS IT YOUR FAULT?

People love to play the blame game but the **undeniable fact**
of the matter is that non-smokers get lung cancer, young
thin active people get diabetes (including Type Two) and
bad things can happen to good people. What matters is not
how you arrived here, what matters is that you're here and
you – yes you and only you – have to make some decisions
about what happens NOW.

I manage one of Australia's most iconic figures, the
original wild man and wildlife warrior Alby Mangels. For
anyone who doesn't know who he is, please go to
albymangels.com, but in brief Alby pioneered the action
adventure reality genre of entertainment with his record-
breaking "World Safari" films, which during one week at
the Sydney Box Office actually out-grossed "Star Wars"!
Alby's die-hard global fan base call him a "dead set
legend" (which is easy to say if you're not trying to manage
someone who has no sense of real time let me tell you) and
a "babe magnet". The point about mentioning Alby here is
that Alby is health obsessive. He has never eaten anything
that isn't organic, low GI, low fat, high fibre, he's never
smoked, rarely drinks, works out every single day and
regularly has all his medical check ups – and you know
what? Even Alby has had medical "issues"… issues that
you wouldn't imagine someone with that lifestyle would
ever have. Sometimes it really is just genetics. You can't
argue with genetics (no matter how much you might like
to) but you can take responsibility for what happens now.

To paraphrase another very wise man, Viktor Frankl, things
will happen to you in your life over which you have no
control but there is one thing you will never lose control of
and that is your ability to choose how you are going to react
to any given situation. As Viktor was an inmate of a Nazi
concentration camp where his entire family was murdered

before his eyes and where he endured grotesque torture and unimaginable pain, both physical and psychological, I think you will have to agree that whatever hardship or trial you may face in your life nothing could conceivably be as dire as what Viktor endured. During his internment Viktor wrote a book in his head called "Man's Search for Meaning", which has since been published and never gone out of print. The point is that you have choices and whatever choice you make you have to take responsibility for – no one is responsible for you, except you.

When Alby and I visited the remote and brutal volcanic island of Tanna in the Vanuatu group with a reporter and photographer from "New Idea" magazine late 2010 (to report on one of our charity missions for the forgotten people of this island who have no medical supplies, no running water and no means of getting their story to the outside world) the four in our group formed a lifelong bond of firm friendship. Since then the forty-something, strappingly good-looking, robustly fit photographer (Andrew) who travelled with us has been diagnosed with inoperable, terminal, lung cancer which has metastasized and spread into the bones. This man has never smoked in his life and has lived following all the right rules. Yet even under this apparent death sentence this man is strong, active and so far he has defied all odds by retaining a positive outlook. He could have wailed, "Why me?" given up and buried his head in denial but instead he is never short of a cheery smile, he's meditating, walking and now he's joined *The Bike Ride to Conquer Cancer*, which I am donating to. Please check out Andrew's new site here which also promotes this book and assists diabetes research too!

www.inspiredaustralians.com

A good attitude and taking responsibility goes a long, long way. We all know the body can do amazing things if the mind will let it, which brings me back to my point about discipline in the "inch by inch" chapter.

We all came back sick, battered and bruised from Tanna… all of us except Alby that is. The reporter, Andrew the photographer and myself had all had our shots, tablets, pills and potions but none of us had Alby's lifetime of experience in the most rugged and unforgiving parts of our planet. After a three hour journey across boulder-strewn, mud-bogged, cliff-edge, hairpin bends into parts of the island no tourist would ever normally travel in order to reach one of these remote villages, we thought we had arrived at our final destination… but no. There was still a forty-five minute climb to reach the village. At the finish, Andrew the photographer (who was in perfect health back then) said, "that was tough", the reporter was carried down by two indigenous islanders puffed beetroot and unable to speak, yet Alby skipped up and back as though he was a mountain goat – and he was thirteen years older than the next eldest in our group (outrageous!) I had fist sized bruises all up and down my arms and legs by the time I returned and later that night I came down with symptoms from eating I don't even want to think what (there was no refusing the hospitality of the chief) but it was worth it all to see the joy and hope we brought to these beautiful island people. However, the point here is how many of them are now dealing with diabetes.

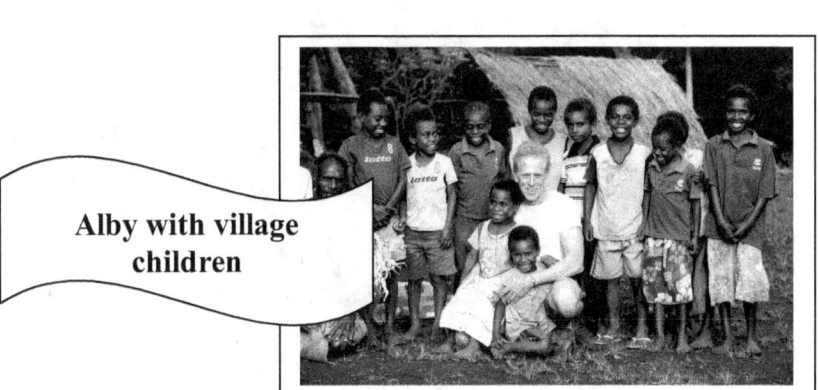

Alby with village children

Well meaning visitors have introduced an otherwise healthy living people to our sugary drinks, processed foods and cigarettes and left their poor unprepared metabolisms to attempt to process these foreign substances. It is not their fault – they don't know any better – we do – we have a choice.

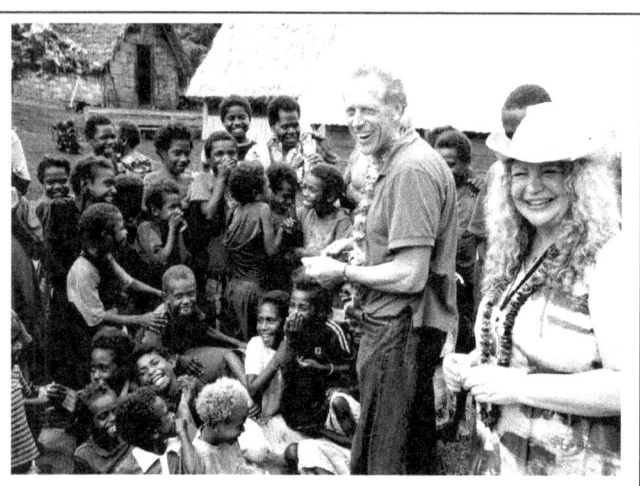

Lynn and Alby teaching the children how to play with a gift of harmonicas

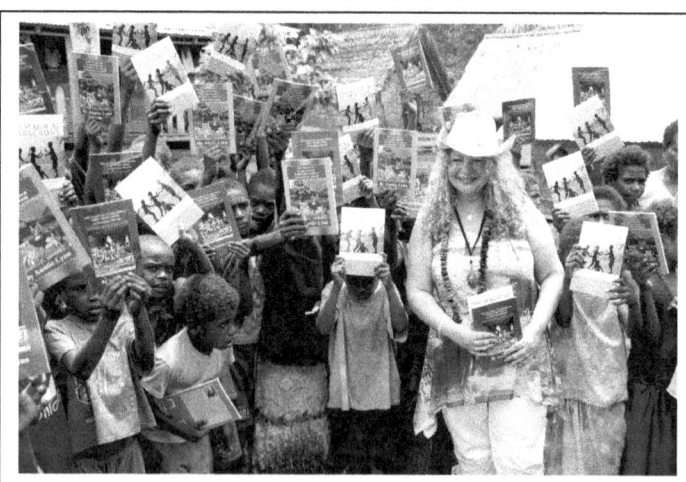

Lynn with a gift of Magical Scarecrows books for the village children

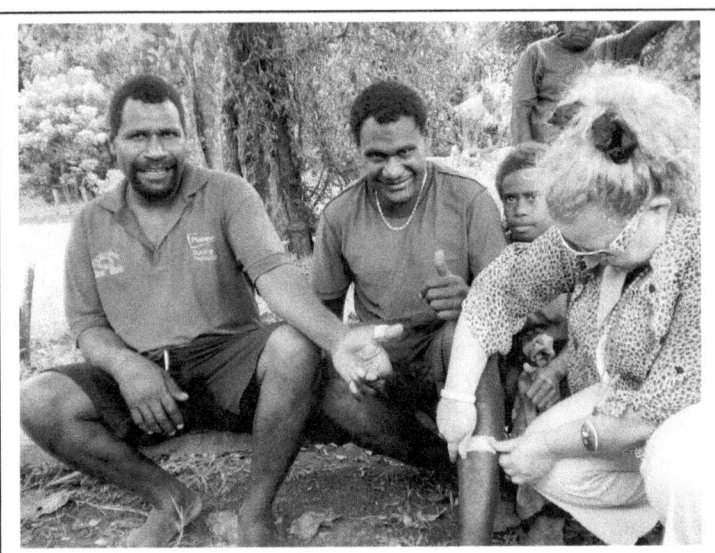

**Nurse Lynn in action with medi powder
and band aids as children watch on…**

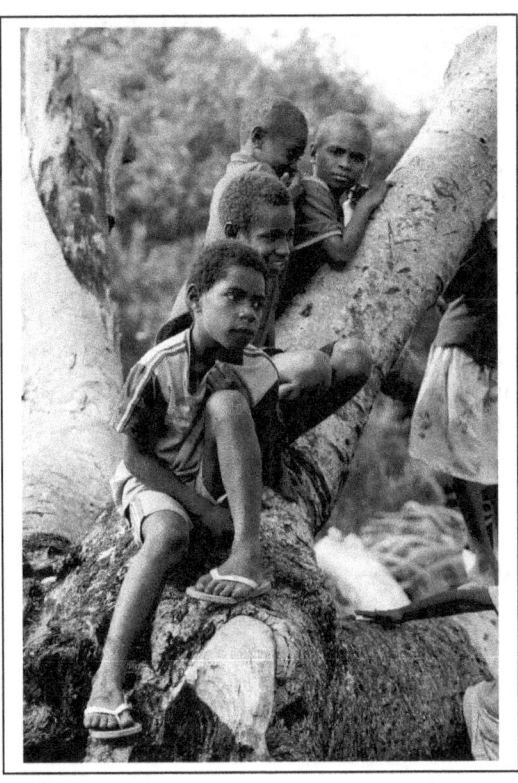

My father had been a model diabetic in almost every way. Coming from the medical background he did perhaps that isn't surprising but I don't think this was truly what motivated him from day one to be a model diabetic. His brother, who was ten years older than my father, was also diagnosed with Type Two diabetes in his mid thirties when he was slim, active and otherwise healthy. My uncle, who was a colourful character by any standard you'd care to measure him, decided as there was no clear and present danger in the form of symptoms manifesting themselves he would live for the day and take no notice of his diabetes. My uncle was dead before his 40th birthday. Let me say that again for any of you who aren't paying attention and think diabetes is not a disease that can kill you – *my uncle ignored his condition and was dead before his 40th birthday.* I hope you are paying attention now!

Perhaps you'll understand why my father, with the benefit of that hindsight and with the benefit of being surrounded by medical experts in his chosen career, was (more or less) a model diabetic. Through good management (eating right and staying active) he remained on oral medication for ten years but even doing everything right once diabetes has established itself it usually persistently progresses. It is what *you* do that will determine whether it progresses at a snail's pace or a thoroughbred gallop. As an insulin requiring diabetic my father continued to do most of the right things for another two decades. Once he retired, the drive to remain physically active seemed to disappear and it wasn't long before his legs were purple from the calves down. Granted he wasn't perfect - my father was a smoker so the purple legs were quite likely as much to do with clogged arteries from smoking as the decline in physical activity. Prolonged heavy smoking will cause the arteries in the leg to clog up and my father smoked from ten years old.

However, smoking issues aside, physical activity is VITAL (for everyone but most especially for people with diabetes) to keep your blood circulating. Even walking 30 minutes a day is enough – that's all you need to do – but ***do it*** – don't let life get in the way of living.

Once the purple legs (and other complications I won't detail) set in with my father that was the beginning of the end. It was a truly terrible and horrendous thing to have witnessed.

In the photos below you will see the size my father was when first diagnosed with type two diabetes (skinny) and below left is only months before the end.

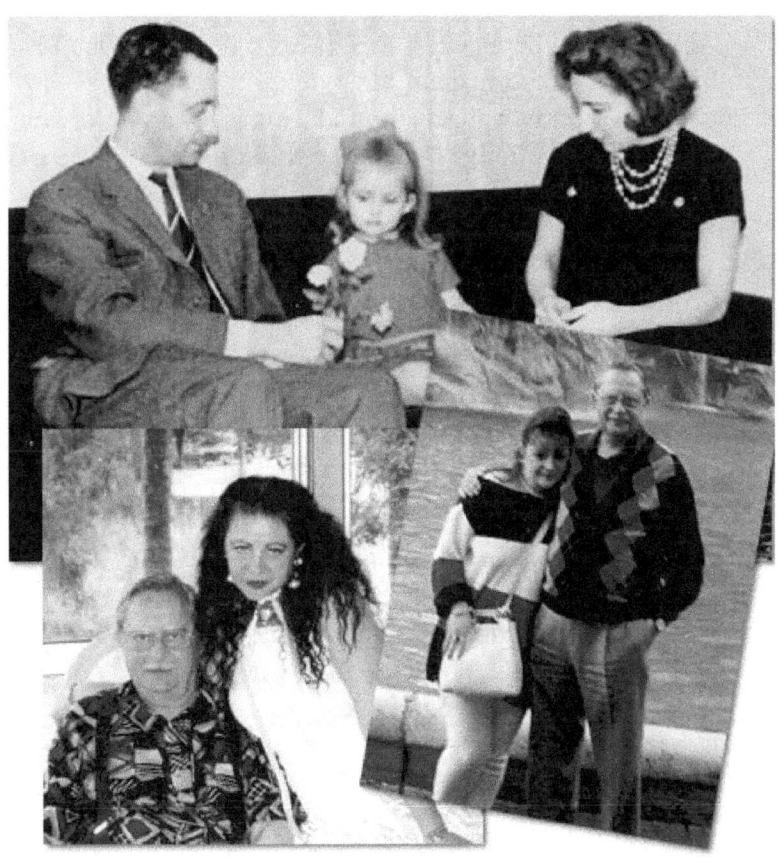

BEATING THE EATING

Okay, keeping to a regimented eating plan can be as irritating as a cactus in your pyjamas but unless we are happy to present all of the mental stability of a bunch of rats in a burning meth lab it is just plain folly not to at least slowly modify our eating habits as diabetics and pre-diabetics… heck everyone can improve their eating habits irrespective of any medical condition. Nobody's perfect and I'm certainly not trying to pretend I am… I tried being patient but it took too long! Your eating regime doesn't have to be regimented but it does have to be sensible and this is where your diabetes dietitian can help.

Weight loss (where necessary) takes time – there isn't a quick fix, it's a permanent lifestyle change. Perhaps some people are happy walking around when they are overweight – although I doubt it. Many in the fashion industry are now trying to address the supersizes with clothes that flatter and disguise as though this new level of normal is acceptable. "They" say it's all about self-esteem. Well, horse hockey! If you want good self-esteem don't disguise your problem – take hold of that sucker head on and beat the living daylights out of it!

Humour is a great way to defuse depression on the surface, but in quiet places that only you see when you turn the light off at night, I wonder how helpful it is then. I recall one large friend shooting back a comment to a person who asked her once, "Don't you think there's a dainty little ballerina in there just trying to get out?" The response? "Only if I ate her and haven't passed her yet!" No doubt that made her feel good in the moment – it was a cool answer – but what about later in the privacy of her own underpants? I wonder how that question played on her mind then.

There are plenty of professionals available to help you. Talk to your GP for a referral to a counsellor and/or a dietitian who specialises in diabetes.

When I first visited my dietitian who specialises in diabetes she was quite astonished at how quickly I'd dropped all the "baddies" from my diet and how organised I'd become with my eating regime. Curious as to how I had managed to get a handle on things so quickly she asked me what had motivated me.

"I've witnessed a diabetic death," I told her solemnly.

A moment's silence passed between us before she replied, "It might be a cruel thing to say, but if everyone I saw had witnessed a diabetic death my job would be a lot easier."

I don't deny I was motivated by fear, knowledge and experience and most people living with diabetes don't have the benefit of these things. There is, of course, no substitute for real experience but I'm going to persist hoping I still have your attention and my little scribblings might just help you down the right path.

Recently I had lunch with Alby Mangels and Lewis Kaplan in Melbourne, during one of Alby's rare and fleeting visits to Australia, to discuss our film project. The subject of Caesar salads came up. Let's just take a quick look at the allegedly healthy Caesar salad:

*   Croutons – white/high GI, fried – bad
*   Dressing – full of saturated fat and sugar – bad
*   Bacon – dripping with saturated fat – bad
The only good thing about a Caesar salad is the lettuce!

If you're trying to eat healthy and at the same time humanely (personally I try never to eat anything that isn't free range – and I've written a lengthy paper for the charity

"Voiceless" as to exactly why) and maybe you're also kosher or halal – well it isn't easy – but it isn't impossible either! The results are worth it. In my first six months as a diagnosed diabetic I lost 12kg without going on a weight loss diet, without compromising my principles for humane eating, without going hungry or feeling I was missing out on anything and keeping strictly to a diabetic eating regime. As a result my first and second three month HbA1c readings came in absolutely text book perfect – yay me!

My own eating regime now consists of three meals a day divided precisely as my dietitian advised, that is 50% green/fibre/vegetables, 25% protein and 25% carbohydrate. That sounds simple so far, but it isn't quite that simple. Some vegetables are much higher in sugar and carbs than others. Carbs can be low GI or high GI. High GI means the sugar content will quickly spike your glucose readings. I could get technical about it, but what's the point? You're not a doctor and neither am I – all you need to know is low GI is good and high GI is bad. White bread and even wholemeal bread is high GI – drop it! Multigrain bread is low GI.

I will explain one thing about spiking your glucose readings. Why is this harmful? Well, as simply as I can put it, if you spike your glucose readings (and some apparently "healthy" options can spike your readings – and I'll talk about well meaning "health farms" later where they are certainly not giving all the right advice – don't think because someone wears a white coat that they know what they're talking about!) but anyway, every time you spike your glucose readings you are putting stress on your pancreas, liver and other bodily tissues (in other words you are causing another notch of irreversible damage).

Make no mistake, diabetes insidiously attacks every cell and organ in your body, even if you're not feeling it happen – and I do mean everything from your eyes to your toes and everything in between. Remember the old weight loss saying, "A moment on my lips – a lifetime on my hips"? well translate that into terms of what you're doing to yourself every time you slip and think of it in terms not of weight gain but bringing forward one of many and varied possible debilitating side effects of the condition and/or more needles required to control it then those tasty bad eating habits might not look quite so appealing any more.

Where protein is concerned it is always better to eat whole food rather than processed (steak rather than hamburgers or sausages, fish rather than fish cakes and so on). White and wholemeal bread are high GI while multigrain bread is low GI, however the carb content varies enormously from one brand to another, so watch out for that. Read labels – read labels – read labels. My mother and I were taught to read labels on everything since I was a small child because of my father's condition, so it's second nature for us, but if you're new to this you need to get into the habit. Do not be taken in by words like "light" or "40% less fat". "Light" can sometimes just refer to the colour! I'll bet you didn't know that! 40% less fat than what? Do not read the marketing messages on the front of products, read the tiny writing on the tables on the back – that's the only way you will know for certain if a product is really safe for you or not. All this impacts your glucose readings. Of course reading labels is one thing but you also need to know what you're looking for on those labels and once again this is where your diabetes dietitian comes into the picture.

Quantities are also important. My personal carb allowance per meal is a potato roughly the size of a large egg but that's what works for me. There is no "one size fits all approach" to diabetes and only your own dietitian can tell you what's right for you. I'm not going to drone on about all the good and bad foods here – there are plenty of other books and people you can go to for advice about that.

Different things are going to work for different people in different circumstances. I will tell you what I do and perhaps some of that will work for you but the best advice is to see a dietitian. My readings are now consistently in the high 4s and 5s (that's around 72 to 90 in the US scale) both before breakfast and two hours after dinner, in fact some of my morning readings have even dropped to the high 3s! I'm positively beside myself (my favourite position) with that result and so is my doctor. Of course those readings are too low for an insulin requiring diabetic as they need to be aware of the risk of hypoglycaemia but they are fabulous for me.

One item now missing from my diet that I miss terribly is cheese. It was eliminated in my initial blitz to bring down my cholesterol reading without taking medication (which will make more sense in a later chapter). I am only mentioning it here to make a point about vegetarian diets (as advocated in some of the "30 day diabetic cures" on the internet and in many health resorts). Let's be clear about something, we are not designed to be vegetarians – we are omnivores. If you want to be vegetarian then full credit to you but as a diabetic you need to be mindful that vegetarian meals are frequently carbohydrate heavy (often with high cheese content). This is not a good option if you are diabetic. Even vegan options are still frequently carbohydrate heavy. When you visit the healthy take-away eatery as opposed to the fried fast food establishment you might feel good about your choice but just take a look at the size of the portions served and how loaded with carbs and cheese they are. You certainly can live well as a vegetarian (and I am not here to try and talk you out of it by any means) but as a diabetic you must watch your carb and saturated fat intake. Just to qualify that point – cholesterol is not something you eat it is already something inside you but foods that contain high levels of saturated fat (like cheese and bacon) will increase your cholesterol levels, which is something to avoid.

Prawns, as an example, do contain cholesterol but cholesterol in food does not affect the cholesterol in our bodies to the same extent as saturated fat (e.g. cheese and bacon).

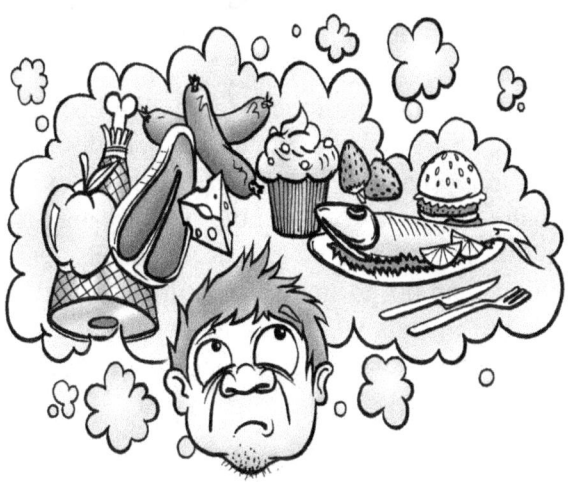

Here's a list of other items now absent from my diet:

- Chocolate (ouch!) although I allow myself one or two squares of sugar free chocolate a day. You have to be careful even there – read the carb and sugar content of the various sugar free chocolate available as some have much higher content than others.
- Crisps/cold chips – completely gone (double ouch!)
- All soft drinks – both fruit juices and fizzy drinks.
- Cointreau on ice (oh the pain! But it's full of sugar.)
- Ice cream (jeepers!) There are sugar free ice creams if you feel the need – thus far, I do not. But once again – check the fat and carb content from one brand to another – they can vary enormously.
- Green Thai Curry (coconut cream is a big "no no" for me), bacon (free range or not – that's out), salami (because it's processed and fatty), white and wholemeal bread, all fast food (no more KFC), chicken skin (which is worse than a bucket of

chips), creamy sauces (which includes many Indian curries), sauces generally (only mustard now – and no salad dressings, just plain Balsamic vinegar.)
- I've reduced the quantity of my carbs – by a lot!
- I have grilled fish instead of crumbed or battered.
- I only use olive oil in cooking (although some other oils are acceptable).

You know what? I loved all these things but because my mind is so focused on pushing back the need for insulin and then risking a hypo and/or becoming blind and/or suffering nerve damage and/or losing a limb… I really and truly don't even miss them. I can watch someone else eating any of these things and not even be tempted. Admittedly I am new to this, but my change of attitude was so instant and profound that I really would be surprised if I reverted back to bad habits – ever.

Fruits contain fructose – or in layman's language – sugar. However, the kind of fruit you eat and what you eat it with all makes a difference. I was quite fascinated to learn from my dietitian that if I cut up a kiwi fruit with my All Bran cereal it lowers the GI absorption of the fruit – cool tip!!

So what do I eat? Well, this is me and what works for me isn't necessarily going to work for you but this is my routine.

If it's a cold breakfast, then All Bran cereal (half a cup) as the fibre. Add a sliced kiwi fruit and a palm full of protein rich nuts (not cashews – they're high in sugars) to the All Bran and use low fat milk. That's the cold breakfast. Hot breakfast could see either yolkless eggs (poached or scrambled – whatever) or a quarter cup of baked beans as the protein, half a bran muffin (the flat kind, not the cake variety) and sautéed tomatoes, spinach and mushrooms in a little olive oil with some ground black pepper. Olive oil (in my opinion) is the healthiest choice in an oil.

Lunch – I love salmon sashimi. I realise that isn't for everyone but I would probably eat this three or four times a week with lettuce and a small quantity of fine Japanese pasta on the side. Please note: that is sashimi and *not* sushi. *Did you know that sushi rice and in fact most Asian dishes are prepared with sugar?* Actually it has been pointed out to me by dietitians at the highly respected Baker Institute that it is not so much the sugar content in sushi rice that is the issue as this is frequently a very low quantity (and not all Japanese restaurants use sugar in their sushi rice) it is more about the carbohydrate in the rice. Many Asian foods do have sugar added to their sauces and the carb content is quite high because of this but the issue with rice (whether white or brown rice) is that it is high GI (yes, brown rice as well). Medium grain rice (jasmine, Arborio, sushi/kwashikori, etc) is high GI. Long grain rice (basmati, doongara, mahatma, wild) are lower GI. If you want to add more fibre to your diet by eating brown rice it is better to eat long grain rice.

Alternatively my lunch could be grilled chicken or fish with coleslaw (where I know the coleslaw dressing is reliable) or green salad or steamed greens. For the carb this can vary between rice, pasta or (horror) I will have some fried chips! Ha – that's my bad… BUT only the tiniest quantity (I literally count out seven chips – depending on the size of the chips). If I'm going out and eating a steak the same side dishes apply and I never have sauces on my steak any more – just Dijon mustard on the side (and no dressing on the salad). It sounds boring but to me it isn't. You have to find your own balance of course. Carbs can also be oven baked or boiled potatoes – at home I weigh those – not more than 50 grams.

Please note, this diet would not suit an insulin requiring diabetic where they need to be aware of the risk of hypoglycaemia but for a Type Two or pre-diabetic on oral or no medication it works very nicely… well it certainly works for me anyway.

Dinner would be vaguely similar to lunch – perhaps grilled salmon – perhaps canned tuna in spring water – perhaps roast beef – that sort of thing for the protein. There are countless varieties of yummy green veggies to choose from and for the carbs more or less the same as lunch.

Snacks – well, I am very careful about snacks. I've never slept much, not since birth, and one of my biggest weaknesses was getting up three or four times in the night and raiding the fridge. Now I find I can't do that without thinking how it's going to affect my morning glucose reading and my three month HbA1c reading – so usually I find myself munching on a piece of cucumber. Fortunately I love cucumbers… and there is no ulterior association with this I assure you! To quote Sigmund Freud, "Sometimes a cigar *really is* just a cigar"!

I always keep some sugar free jelly made up in the fridge for "emergencies" – I find that doesn't impact my readings at all. I will allow myself one or two squares of the lowest carb/sugar content "sugar free" chocolate per day.

NOTE:
None of the "sugar free" chocolates are free of all sugars – always read the table on the back. And FYI – medications, particularly cough mixtures, are often loaded with sugar!

TIP:
Take your reading glasses (if you wear them) with you when you go shopping. It's no accident that tables displaying sugar, fat and carb content on the back of food products are written by miniature magical elves!!!

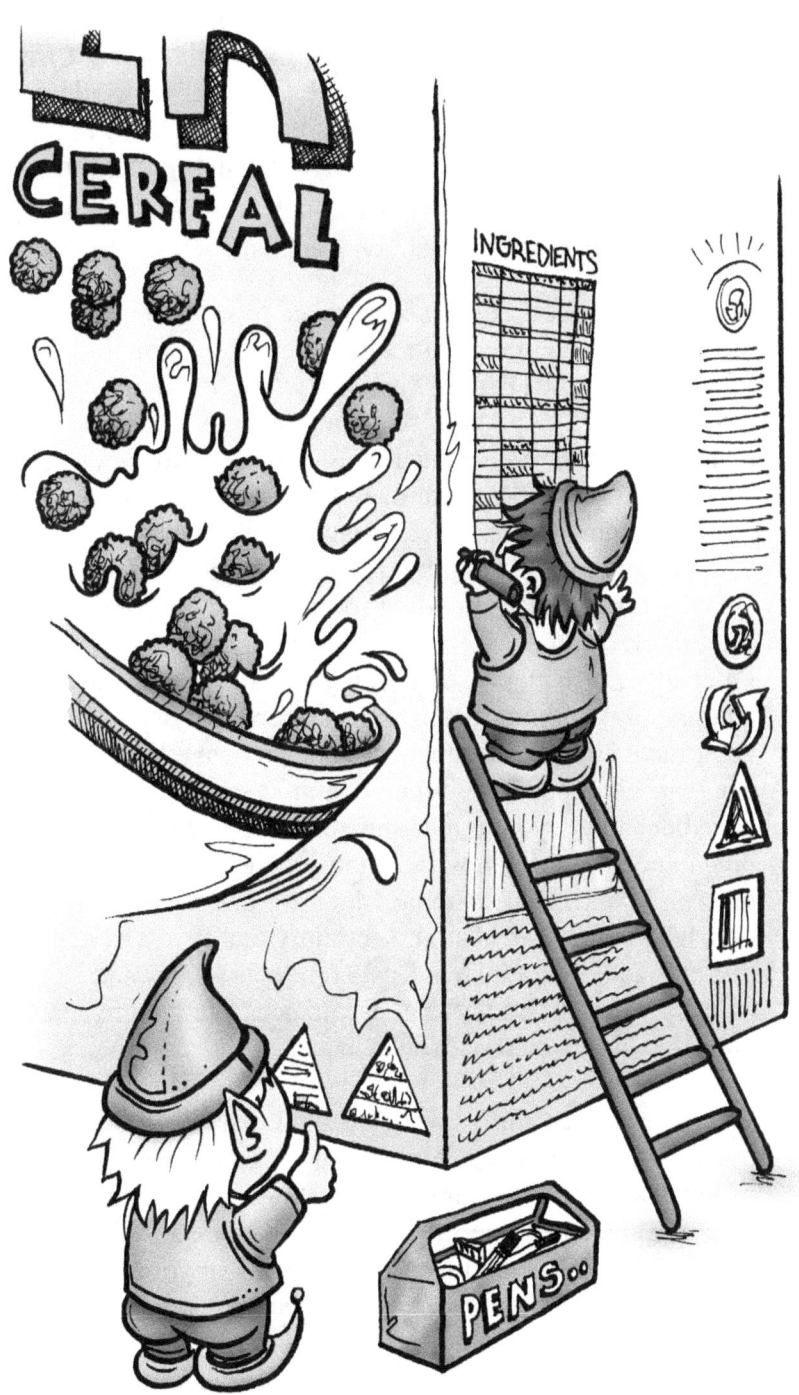

What I have not cut out is my after dinner glass of *dry* wine (or two or three glasses of wine when I socialise) and if I'm going to be totally honest (hoping this doesn't blow all my credibility with my readers) I still smoke. Shocking, I know, but I've cut my intake down to ten a day and, for now, that's just going to have to do. See – I told you I wasn't perfect!

A word on smoking I have been asked to include by Professor Paul Zimmet from the Baker International Diabetes Institute (Paul is frowning at me for admitting I smoke at all). The point of this book (as opposed to the myriad of other dry, technical publications on diabetes) is that (a) it is very openly frank and personal and (b) I am admitting I am an imperfect, flawed, real person - just like you. No one is going to get it all right - we are not perfect creatures. Just because I admit to smoking does not make it right or clever or acceptable or any less dangerous - especially for diabetics. This is my bad and perhaps it's a whopper but without making excuses or justifying my bad habit there have been many smokers who have lived to old age (ask Winston Churchill and countless others) and there have been many young non-smokers who have contracted lung cancer (ask Andrew the photographer and countless others). Smoking is a gamble, albeit I grant you a stupid one, whereas it is an absolute certainty that if you have diabetes and do not take at least some steps to try and manage your condition the consequences *will* be dire and once they occur there is no way back.

The point is everything GOOD you do will help your overall wellbeing and as I said in the beginning, the journey of a thousand miles begins with the first step. Even if you take one piece of advice away from this book it will be one positive thing you are doing for yourself that you weren't doing before - and kudos to you for that! Eating right, daily exercise and maintaining the daily, quarterly and annual check ups are a major part of good management.

MANY DIFFERENT DIETS WORK

I found this to be quite fascinating stuff. It was Professor Paul Zimmet, Director Emeritus of the prestigious and highly regarded Baker International Diabetes Institute, who suggested I look into it. Paul is an amazing man with a remarkable and esteemed background. He is also a good friend of a very good friend of mine and my late father's (which is how we started talking) and it turns out that Paul's mentor in diabetes was none other than my own father's diabetic specialist! Small world! Paul very reasonably suggested that different lifestyles are suited to different diets and you would be well advised to discuss with your dietitian which (out of many) diets suits your particular lifestyle. There are many to choose from! For example: vegetarian, Mediterranean, glycemic index and even traditional "hunter-gatherer" diets (or at least the modern version thereof).

The **Paleolithic diet** popularly referred to as the **caveman diet**, **Stone Age diet** and **hunter-gatherer diet**, is a modern nutritional plan based on the presumed ancient diet of wild plants and animals that various hominid species habitually consumed during the Paleolithic era. Centred on commonly available modern foods, the "contemporary" Paleolithic diet consists mainly of fish, grass-fed pasture raised meats, vegetables, fruit, fungi, roots and nuts, and excludes grains, legumes and dairy products. A common theme in evolutionary medicine, Paleolithic nutrition is based on the premise that modern humans are genetically adapted to the diet of their Paleolithic ancestors and that human genetics have scarcely changed since the dawn of agriculture therefore an ideal diet for human health and well-being is one that resembles this ancestral diet.

Those in favour of this diet argue that modern human populations subsisting on traditional diets similar to those of Paleolithic hunter-gatherers are largely free of the diseases of modern civilization and have shown some positive health outcomes regardless of whether a high percentage of dietary energy is supplied by wild animal foods (e.g. in Canadian Eskimos), wild plant foods (e.g. in the Kung), or domesticated plant foods (e.g. in the Yanomamo).

Food has played a major role in human evolution but in a somewhat different manner than is generally appreciated. Humans are not self-made creations dietarily but rather have an evolutionary history as anthropoid primates stretching back more than 25 million years. Hunter-gatherers were not free to determine their diets, rather it was their predetermined biological requirements for particular nutrients that constrained their evolution. I said before I am not going to take on the role of dietitian in this book but this is a fascinating area it is well worth you taking further in discussions with your specialist/s.

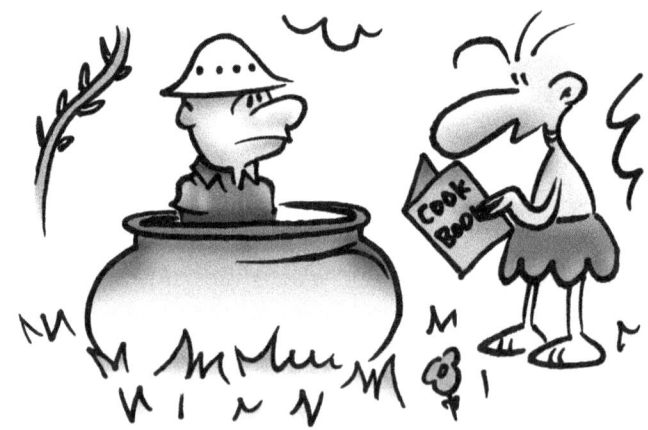

"TRADITIONAL HUNTER — GATHERER DIET???"

THE SOCIAL ANIMAL

Eating out, socialising, travelling and attending events can be tricky. Many of my fellow diabetics don't like to identify themselves as diabetics for fear they will be seen as odd, difficult, or challenging to accommodate. As I have no problem whatsoever in being seen as odd, difficult, or challenging to accommodate it poses no problem for me! But that's me – everyone is different. In my brief time as a diabetic I quickly discovered there are restaurants where diabetics are not catered for at all, airline food can pose a major problem, parties frequently offer little by way of suitable sustenance for a diabetic diet and at an event you can be trapped into eating only what is served when it is served. If you really are trapped then the world won't stop spinning if you eat the wrong food on a rare occasion but please try to be mindful and plan ahead. Make people you are going to socialise with, or an airline you are going to travel with, aware in advance of your condition and requirements. If you don't stand up for yourself who is going to do it for you? Generally I have found people to be very accommodating and understanding – even interested.

As I stated earlier, it is always better to get all the nutrients you need through diet rather than pills (better for you – not so good for the pill manufacturers of course) and it is always better to lower your glucose levels (when necessary) through physical activity rather than medication (where possible). I have been advised that if you absolutely must have that piece of chocolate cake on a *very rare* occasion then you will need to up your medication to compensate but don't make a habit of it because this *will* spike your readings. If that piece of chocolate cake was consumed at a party or celebration dinner the chances are you'll be heading home with your partner afterwards and let's not forget that physical activity comes in all shapes and sizes. Sex will bring your readings down and it's not bad exercise to get the blood circulating too!

Okay, I'm being glib, but the point I'm making is that sex will lower your glucose readings so be mindful of this fact.

You do not have to compromise lifestyle to be a good diabetic, but if you are a bad diabetic I guarantee you *will* be compromising lifestyle – if not life.

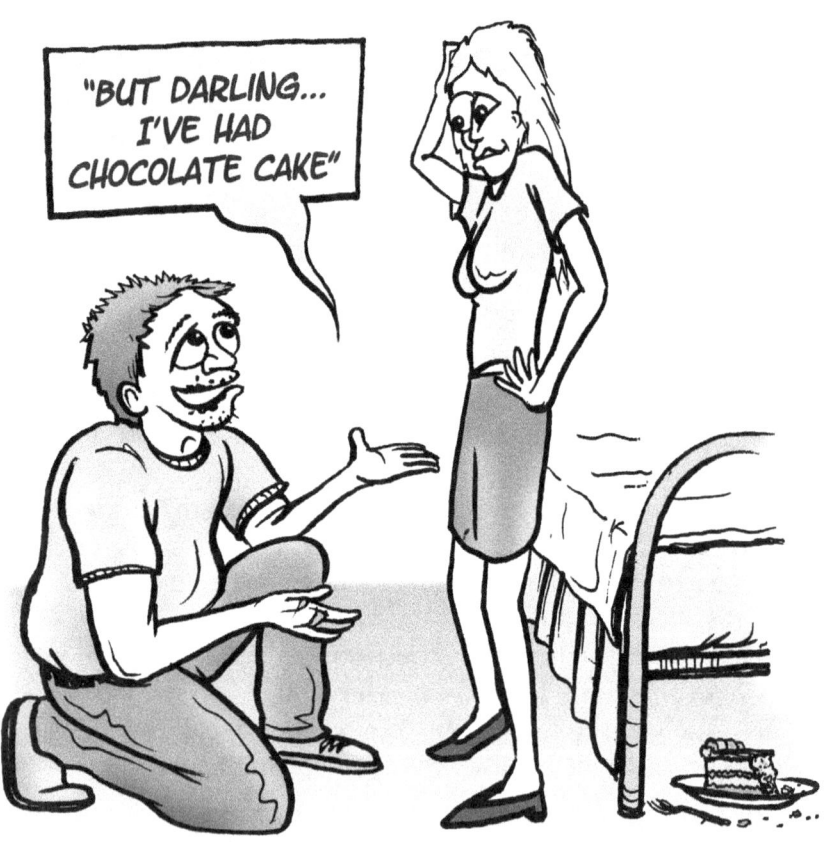

Along the lines of standing up for yourself I am going to share with you some dialogue I have had with a major airline and a major health resort.

Without naming the particular airline, let's just say the brand name would probably not reflect the status of any woman that Alby has come in contact with, indeed that might in fact be **verging** on the ridiculous.

You have important dietary requirements that must be adhered to – say it loud and say it clear. The more of us who do so, the more likely public places and services are to pay attention – that's people power! It's your life at stake, so don't be shy in asking for that which you require and deserve, as I did...

Dear xxxxxxxxx,

Further to my original email on this matter I have since flown twice in business class with your airline and have been appalled to the point of being devastated at the complete lack of consideration given to your diabetic passengers. In Australia there are over a million diagnosed diabetics (Type One and Two) and almost that number again who have not been diagnosed, plus two million pre-diabetics. On both my recent flights there was nothing I was able to eat served in the business class cabin. I had asked in advance to make a special dietary request and was told this was not offered on your domestic flights – under any circumstances – but a food voucher would be offered if the meal of choice was not available. One cannot eat a food voucher and diabetics must eat certain foods at prescribed times.

On my first flight I was offered afternoon tea comprised of a raspberry tart, quince jam, grapes which contain an extremely high sugar content, cheese which is high in cholesterol which is damaging to diabetics and to add insult to injury when I asked for something as simple as a cup of green tea I discovered that your variety of green tea is infused with pear, another fruit that is high in fructose content.

On the return flight I was flying over lunchtime and the two meals served in the business class cabin were a pasta dish that contained only carbohydrate (whereas a diabetic should have a combination of carbohydrate plus protein plus salad, vegetables or other greens) and a prawn curry. The pasta dish also had a sauce that could have contained any manner of unsafe ingredients for a diabetic. As for the prawn curry, prawns contain cholesterol, not to mention once again the curry sauce could have contained (and almost certainly did) any number of ingredients a diabetic needs to avoid. On this occasion I was fortunate to find one item on the economy menu suitable for my diet, but this both deprived me of a hot meal on a cold day and once again deprived me of a business class meal that I had paid for.

I look forward to your swift attention to this matter and in the meantime remain…

Yours faithfully,
Lynn Santer

Dear Ms Santer

Thank you for taking the time to forward your feedback regarding your experience with us. We appreciate that you have provided us with your valuable comments and concerns.

I sincerely apologise for the lack of diabetic food and snacks on our menu. We regularly assess our in-flight menu and certainly take into account the feedback received from our valued guests when these decisions are made. It certainly is concerning to hear that we have no food suitable for you to enjoy during your flight with us. I have been in contact with my catering colleagues and they have advised me that we are currently exploring the options of placing these types of meals onboard. While I'm unable to give a time frame at this stage I will keep you up to date with the progress.

In closing, I once again thank you for forwarding your feedback and I do hope that we have the chance to welcome you back on board in the near future in order to rectify the poor impression gained.

Kind regards

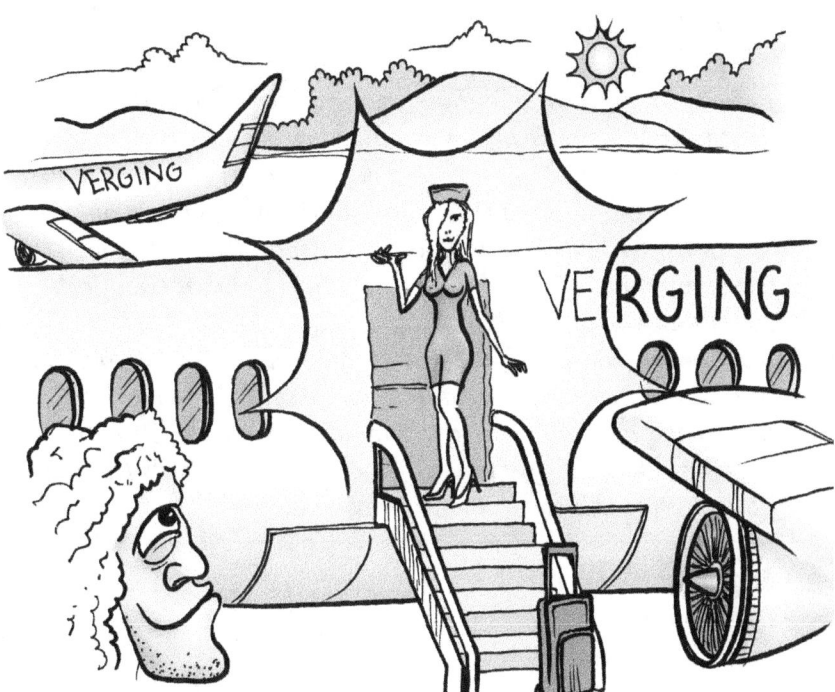

Yes, I do keep every single piece of correspondence both inbound and outbound. If you'd like to see the more amusing emails hop onto my website: **lynnsanter.com** and hit "new release" where you'll find a title called ***Emails from the Edge*** – a book I published after many friends (who had dubbed me "the email queen") begged me to put a compilation together.

This next email trail has been massively edited (axed) as I'd rather not be sued by the first health farm I really took to task after they displayed absolutely no willingness whatsoever to accommodate my diabetic diet. Rather than include the tirade of emails that flowed back and forth between a lady I have dubbed "silly Shirley" and myself I will just share with you the final one with the attachment from a health resort who really did get it right.

Dear Shirley,

Please see below the written response just received from another health resort. This is how a health resort should be run – showing respect, intelligence and consideration both for a controlled diabetic and for good customer and public relations. Only after I had both corresponded and spoken with personnel in the other facility did I tell them about the communications that have transpired between us. They were horrified at both the lack of respect shown to a person who has their condition under control and the completely dismissive attitude of making any attempt whatsoever to accommodate my specific requests. This is not exactly the attitude you will see in the response below.

Sincerely,
Lynn Santer

Dear Lynn

Following our discussion regarding your dietary requirements I would like to confirm a number of points.

Firstly congratulations for having achieved such successful control over your diabetes and maintaining stable blood sugar levels through a strict dietary regime! Well done.

I understand you will require breakfast at 6am and to achieve this we can provide you with either a gluten free muesli (as it has limited dried fruit, which we discussed you would be happy to pick out) with low fat milk or a porridge variety that may be prepared easily in your room. In order to achieve this it would be useful to collect your breakfast from the restaurant staff the night prior - if this arrangement is suitable then we will organise that on arrival. You may then attend tai chi at 6.30am and participate in the activity classes run by our program staff should you choose.

Breakfast for all guests is at 8am and it would be lovely if you could join us for breakfast, even if you do not eat anything further at this time, so long as this won't upset you, as this is an important part of the bonding part of our program and a chance to get to know our staff and fellow guests.

Morning tea may certainly be a small orange – this is served at 10.30am and would be labelled with your name. If there are any other fruit varieties you desire then please feel free to let me know and I can plan for that.

Afternoon tea is served at 3.30pm and is a small serve of nuts and seeds (there may be a very small amount of dried fruit that you could discard or we can arrange for the kitchen staff to put together a small serve sans dried fruit). We often have muffins however they are sweetened with fruit juice or fresh fruit and may not be suitable so again please let me know if you can think of alternatives I can plan around.

Lunch is served at 1pm and dinner at 6pm – once your booking is confirmed I will ask the chefs to put together a current menu plan that you may review and inform me of any ingredients you feel should be deleted from your meals. If the meal does not require significant alterations there will be no further charge, however should there be anything requiring major change there will be a $10 per meal surcharge as we have quite a small kitchen brigade.

We regularly cater to vegetarians, vegans, seafood allergies and nut allergies and anything outside this is usually charged at the nominal rate above.

Please feel free to communicate with me should you have any further concerns / queries, happy to go over the menu with you in detail and plan your meals to allow you to maintain those wonderful readings.

Thanks Lynn, look forward to hearing from you soon.

Kind regards,
Name deleted
Operations Manager

If you want to know which resorts are getting it right and which are getting it wrong (that I know of... according to the Lynn Santer litmus test) drop me a line and ask!

One final note on standing up for yourself. I was recently taken to dinner by a very good friend of mine who is a retired homicide detective (and now a high-flying barrister) who happens to love gourmet food. Have you ever tried saying "no" to either a homicide detective or a high-flying barrister? It is not an easy proposition, let me assure you! There was almost nothing on the menu at this fancy restaurant that was suitable for me to eat. Eventually I settled on a fish dish but even that turned up with a suspicious looking sauce. When I queried the chef as to what was in the sauce he asked me why I wanted to know. I explained that I am a diabetic. He proudly assured me there was no sugar. Well, that was nice but not good enough. I wanted to know what else was in the sauce and it turned out to be loaded with nuts – which are fine if you haven't already got a plate loaded with sufficient quantities of protein and carbs, but when you do they will tip you over the edge of acceptable limits. I left the sauce. The chef was offended. I lost no sleep over this fact and my readings that night were once again perfect.

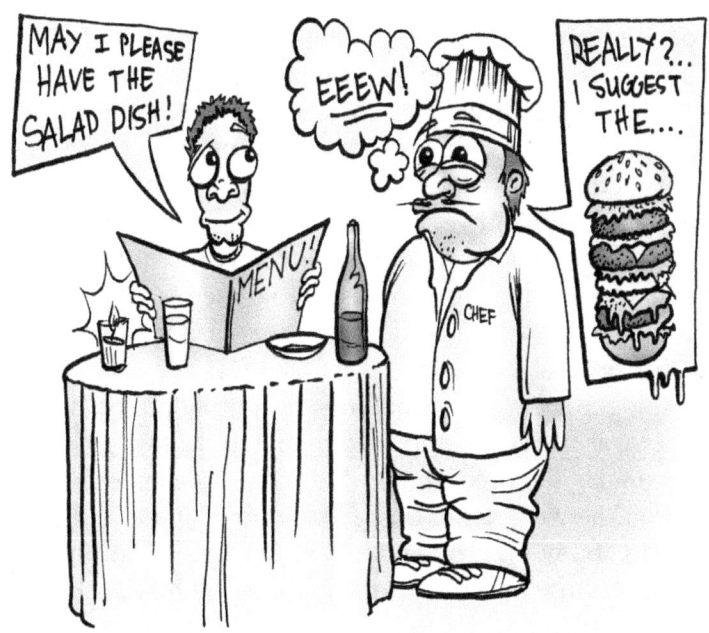

WELL MEANING FRIENDS

One of the hardest things to deal with as a diabetic is well-meaning friends. No one wants to offend those special people in our lives and none of us want to become social pariahs by becoming too difficult to feed at a relaxed gathering of the nearest and dearest. I know I have spoken about what to do if you absolutely have to have that piece of chocolate cake on a ***very rare*** occasion but if you are blessed with a large circle of friends who like to invite you to their homes on a regular basis that doesn't qualify as a very rare occasion. If you start making a habit of saying, "It's only once" and "I feel fine" and "it doesn't matter just for today" then you will be hastening on the day when those insulin injections are going to be necessary to keep you alive, hastening on the day when your legs aren't working as well as they should be, hastening on the day when suddenly you find your eyesight isn't functioning as well as it could be for someone of your age and frankly you'll be hastening on the day of your death.

Every single day, every single thing you eat – and drink – affects your diabetes and by consequence your wellbeing and longevity. Every time I consume anything I always think, "How is this going to impact my next reading?" It might seem overly cautious for a newly diagnosed Type Two diabetic on only one tablet a day but the point is I aim to keep that status for as long as humanly possible. A casual acquaintance of mine sadly told me recently that her son was diagnosed with diabetes a few years ago when he was fifteen years old. To start with he was very good at managing it and as the condition was in the family his mother was already familiar with how to deal with the situation. By the time her son had turned seventeen, however, he was sick of being "abnormal", he felt fine, said, "to hell with it" and started to live like a "normal" person. Within a year he had neuropathy in his leg. His leg will now be painful for the rest of his life – the condition is irreversible – once the damage is done, it's done. He's back on track now and understands that he can't let his vigilance slip if he's going to live a long, pain free, happy life but it took a harsh lesson to make him realise this fact.

Just recently I was invited by one of the many beautiful and wonderful friends I have been blessed with to a social gathering. I had guessed in advance this was going to be a culinary challenge for me so I had my main meal and my medication at lunchtime (instead of dinner time as usual). I was not wrong. When I arrived and saw what was laid out on the table there was nothing I could eat except some cut up cucumber and celery. There were no less than three diabetics at the table – one of whom was the husband of the hostess!

"Try the chicken," my hostess urged me. "It's coated in Ritz crackers."

Now an occasional Ritz cracker is fine but I'd seen these chicken pieces marinating before they were coated and cooked, so I enquired what they had been soaking in.

"Buttermilk," she told me proudly. "There's no sugar in buttermilk."

I really do appreciate the extra effort taken to make food interesting and well presented but for the sake of a strict diabetic, as she knew me to be, what's wrong with simple herbs and spices where there is no risk of sugar or carbs? Aside from that, commercial buttermilk is sweet (see across) and just take a look at the tiny chart written by miniature magical elves on the back of a buttermilk container and check out the fat and carbohydrate content. This extract on buttermilk is taken from The National Centre for Biotechnological Information in their "Composition of Foods" section:

Buttermilk is a dairy ingredient widely used in the food industry because of its emulsifying capacity and its positive impact on flavour. **Commercial buttermilk is sweet** *buttermilk, a by-product from churning sweet cream into butter. However, other sources of buttermilk exist, including cultured and whey buttermilk obtained from churning of cultured cream and whey cream, respectively. The compositional and functional properties (protein solubility, viscosity, emulsifying and foaming properties) of sweet, sour and whey buttermilk were determined at different pH levels and compared with those of skim milk and whey. Composition of sweet and cultured buttermilk was similar to skim milk and composition of whey buttermilk was similar to whey, with the exception of* **fat content, which was higher in buttermilk than in skim milk** *or whey* **(6 to 20% vs. 0.3 to 0.4%).** *Functional properties of whey buttermilk were independent of pH, whereas sweet and cultured buttermilk exhibited lower protein solubility and emulsifying properties as well as a higher viscosity at low pH (pH <or= 5). Sweet, sour and whey buttermilks showed higher emulsifying properties and lower foaming capacity than milk and whey because of* **the presence of milk fat globule membrane components.** *Furthermore, among the various buttermilks, whey buttermilk was the one showing the highest emulsifying properties and the lowest foaming capacity. This could be due to a higher ratio of phospholipids to protein in whey buttermilk compared with cultured or sweet buttermilk. Whey buttermilk appears to be a promising and unique ingredient in the formulation of low pH foods.*

And then came… the CAKE.

"But it's all low fat and fake sugar," I was told.

Hum, okay, let's take a look at that for a moment. Sure enough our charming hostess had used "fake sugar" and the lowest fat possible cream cheese in making this cheese cake. Without going into the other ingredients in the cake itself let's consider to start with the half inch thick crumbed biscuit base (just imagine the carb and sugar content to consider there, or even just the carb content if – "if" – the biscuits used were sugar "free") and then there was the topping.

"But the topping is one of those French jams with no added sugar," she told me.

Alright, let's just review that wording… "no **added** sugar." All fruit has fructose (that's another word for sugar) and again check out the tiny table on the jar written by the miniature magical elves and you'll see there is still sugar content in jams that have no "added" sugar. Even if there was zero sugar in the cake it still had carb and calorie content to consider. Had I eaten one slice of this cheesecake and nothing else I can guarantee I would not have achieved my nightly reading of 4-5 (that's around 72 to 90 in the US scale). Now not all diabetics aim to keep their readings that low, most are happy with readings around 7 (that's around 126 in the US scale) and if you are an insulin requiring diabetic you should be aiming for readings around 7 two hours after eating. However, I have made a conscious decision to keep my readings as low as possible for all the reasons previously stated.

Another person at the table sort of rolled his eyes at me and scoffed, "But you're only on one tablet a day – that's practically not diabetic at all – why do you even care?" The comment would have been disturbing enough in its own right but what made it more disturbing was that this man's son is diabetic. The son was one of those who was diagnosed as Type Two when he was in his thirties, trim and active. The son had adopted the attitude just espoused by his father and quickly his diabetes all but spiralled out of control. He is on multiple insulin injections and numerous tablets every day just to keep him alive. If I needed any justification for my stand point his very own son was living proof of exactly why you take this condition seriously from day one – ***every day*** - forever! I watched my father die from diabetes. I sat at his side as he took his last breath. I know what this disease can do. As I've said, I'm not perfect, not by a long shot. I would not profess to be doing everything right but if it's a choice of not offending a friend and eating food I know is bad for me or pushing off the terrible things I know can happen to me… well to me it's not much of a choice at all.

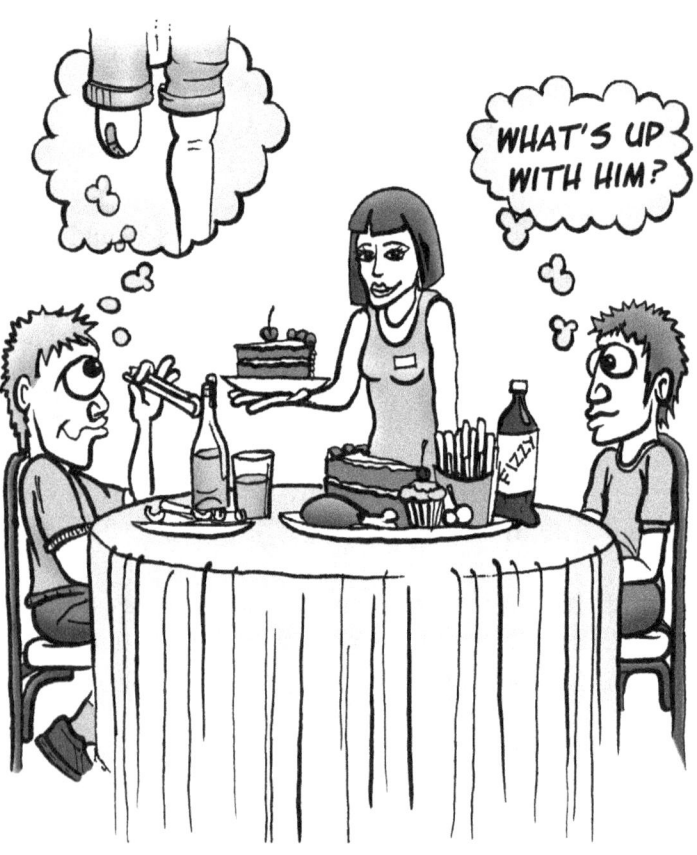

My friends also couldn't understand why I didn't drink as much champagne as they had become accustomed to seeing me drink, or why I left early to return home and eat food I knew was safe for my very strict diet. To me it was quite clear. When I looked around the table (Jarlsberg cheese – high fat/high cholesterol; dips and chips – even if the dips were low fat/no sugar, I said "if", the chips definitely weren't low fat and were most likely cooked in Canola oil as most chips are… and Canola oil is the highest in cholesterol you can get in an oil; cashew nuts – the highest sugar and GI you can get in a nut; pâté – high fat/high cholesterol, not to mention I have a moral objection to eating anything that has been produced from force-feeding hapless animals; assorted fruits – the strawberries were okay, even though one still has to account for their fructose content they are lower than some other fruits, but the other fruits were all very high in sugar content, especially the grapes; the aforementioned chicken; and the aforementioned cheesecake) there was no possible way of having my 25% whole and unadulterated protein, 25% low GI carb and 50% wholesome greens or veg for my dinner at this table – none. Still, I ate a few sticks of celery, drank no less than two glasses of champagne, had a laugh, exchanged some gossip, gave everyone a hug and returned to the sanctuary of my home. It's your life – it's your choice – what will you do?

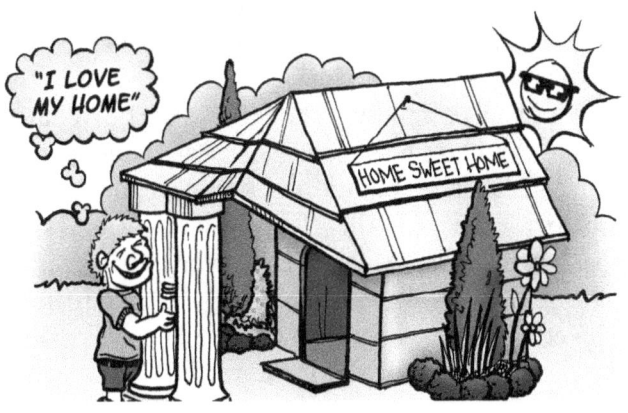

DON'T FEEL LIKE A PRICK?

In the introduction I explained *how* I came up with the title for this book and the film that Alby and I are co-producing in collaboration with Diabetes Australia, but not *why* I chose that title.

"Don't feel like a prick?" means different things to different people.

To Lewis Kaplan (CEO of Diabetes Australia) it means diabetics are sick of sticking themselves with needles (lancets) several times a day to check their glucose readings (I can relate to that!!)

To my diabetic doctor it means diabetics on oral medication are terrified of having to move to insulin injections multiple times a day.

To me it means people are frightened to have a blood test to find out if they have diabetes or not.

And to Alby it means – don't be idiot and do what has to be done.

The film "Don't feel like a prick?" (a question, not a statement) is designed to encourage people to get tested because there are so many undiagnosed diabetics and pre-diabetics walking around in our society blissfully unaware of the ticking time bomb inside them just waiting to explode. I was completely shocked when I explained this to my doctor and he said to me, "What do diabetics fear most? Blindness? Limb amputation? Coma? Death?" According to my doctor the thing they fear most is – needles! My eyes almost came out on stalks like a cartoon character but according to his experience this was the biggest fear. However, now I have had the chance to speak with many specialists in the field who have treated thousands of patients over decades the more robust consensus is a fear of all those things: blindness, limb amputation, coma, death... and needles! Yet still only 18% of diagnoses diabetes have a chronic disease management program in place!

Three people very close to me were each diagnosed with Type Two diabetes in recent years. At that time they were all in their thirties or forties, they were all trim and they were all active. On top of that two of them had no history of diabetes in their family. They all knew my father and all knew he was an insulin requiring diabetic, but my beloved late father was a very private man and only presented himself to friends when he was at his very best. Hence none of these people ever saw what went on behind closed doors and how serious his condition was. Two of these three people (we'll call them Arthur and Martha) did not take their condition as seriously as they could, or should, have. They continued to eat whatever they pleased and believed popping a pill would just keep everything under control. Both Arthur and Martha are now on multiple insulin injections a day, they have both suffered one of the most frightening side-effects for an insulin requiring diabetic – the hypoglycaemic low – and both have said if they had their time over they would have done things very differently. Unfortunately once the damage is done it is irreversible. If you are a newly diagnosed Type Two diabetic, or pre-diabetic – heed these words because otherwise soon this could be you! 40-50% of Type Two diabetics will have to move onto insulin sooner or later but the better you manage your condition the longer you can push this off.

There are many instances where insulin production fails through no fault of the person - this is not curable and not reversible and the reason why daily and quarterly and annual checks are imperative.

Good management of your diabetes does not necessary mean you will stay off insulin as there are instances where your pancreas will fail eventually but the better you manage your condition the less likely this is to occur and the further you can push that likelihood back. If you do not manage your condition it pretty much guarantees you will end up on insulin, heighten your risk of neuropathy and potential limb amputation, heighten your risk of retinopathy and losing your eyesight, increase the likelihood of the onset of multiple daily injections and the thing that is associated with this and terrifies me the most - the risk of hypoglycaemic lows.

The third friend, we'll call him Jason, took his condition very seriously from day one. For nine years, let me say that again – *nine years* – he kept his condition under control with diet and exercise alone. Only recently has he moved onto one oral tablet per day whereas in less time the other two have had to start sticking themselves with multiple needles on a daily basis. Not everything that happens is your choice – but some of what happens is. Choose today – choose now – that you are going to be the person who takes responsibility and ownership for managing your condition and you will be grateful for the rest of your (hopefully) very long and healthy life.

While we're on the subject of pricks, here's another mistake almost all newly diagnosed diabetics make – they don't take their glucose readings regularly. Too many don't even get their three monthly (HbA1C) blood tests done and those who do think the three monthly average is enough of a gauge so they don't need to prick themselves twice or more a day to see what's going on. Wrong! Why? I'll tell you…

If you don't take your readings before you eat in the morning and two hours after you eat at night (at least) and record what you've been eating, how much you've exercised and what your readings were as a result, you are never going to get on top of understanding what are the right combinations of food and activity for you. There is no one size fits all with diabetes – this is the *only* way to know for certain what works best for you.

Please see the easy reference chart on page 95 to use as a guide.

TIP:

I kinda wish my doctor had told me this before we discussed me writing this book, but better late than never. Pricking the pads of your fingers twice a day or more hurts – let's not pretend otherwise. Both as a writer and as a pianist I spend a good portion of my life on one keyboard or another. My hands are very literally my life and having sore fingertips all the time was dang depressing. Well, guess what… you don't need to prick the pads of your fingers – prick the sides where there are far less nerve endings. I've been doing that ever since I was told and while you still fleetingly feel the swift prick, there is no residual soreness afterwards! Brilliant!

This same doctor doesn't want me to talk about my young, thin, active friends and family who have been diagnosed with Type Two diabetes and he certainly doesn't want me to talk about four other friends of mine who respectively weigh in between 140kg – 200kg – none of whom are even pre-diabetic (they've all been tested) and all of whom have perfect cholesterol readings – in fact the only people I know who have cholesterol readings in the double digits are skinny. It's true! I understand why he doesn't want me to say this but while my tiny selection of friends and family may not be at all representative of the overall statistics in Australia, or the world, they are representative of my little corner of the world and after discussions with other experts in the field it isn't as uncommon as you might suppose to find young, thin, active people diagnosed with Type Two diabetes (notwithstanding please cross reference the chapter on Latent Autoimmune Diabetes in Adults).

Of course being morbidly obese (and 140kg – 200kg is definitely morbidly obese) is not healthy even if you have thus far managed to escape diabetes and high cholesterol – it is putting a strain on your heart, it is damaging your joints and just ask yourself how many eighty year old people you see who are overweight. If you're overweight start losing weight – now. It is not acceptable, it is not healthy and it certainly isn't pretty – sorry, but this isn't a book about pulling punches.

The point about making this point is that whether the doctors like me saying it or not, not every overweight person is going to become diabetic and not every young, thin, active person is going to be granted a free pass. Sometimes bad things happen to good people – it's a fact of life. I understand another reason why doctors might not like me saying that thin and active people can get Type Two diabetes is because then what possible motive is there for you to be your ideal weight and physically active if bad things can happen to you anyway? It's a reasonable question – and here's the answer…

If you are your ideal weight and physically active and otherwise healthy and sadly you still are diagnosed with an illness or ailment, you will be far better placed to cope with and fight off that condition if your body is otherwise functioning at peak efficiency. If you have a fatty liver, enlarged heart, clogged arteries, high cholesterol, high blood pressure and/or poor circulation (and all overweight people do have one or more of those conditions) you don't stand much of a chance of fighting off anything. You can try and disguise it all you like with clever clothes and cosmetic enhancements, but even if you're hit by more lasers than the Star Ship Enterprise, your body is still going to know the truth. The photographer, Andrew, I spoke about earlier who has thus far defied all medical predictions would not still be watching his son grow up and enjoying tender moments with his loving wife if his body didn't give him a chance to fight back in the beginning.

So I'm sorry... no wait... no I'm not... I'm not sorry at all for saying thin and active people can get sick too – but that doesn't mean you shouldn't aspire to be the best that you can be... for your own sake... for the sake of those who love you... and for the sake of achieving whatever it is you've been put on this earth to achieve. Don't let your apathy or denial prevent you from living to your pre-destined expiry date – get out there and grab life with both hands and give it all you've got. Everyone, please, go and get pricked once a year. It's only sensible advice to have your annual health checks, no matter what age or size you are, so don't dither, dawdle or procrastinate – just do it.

Up to sixty percent of pre-diabetics *can* turn their condition around by losing weight and exercising, which by definition also means forty percent cannot. But even if you are in that forty percent you can start to manage and control the condition, keeping at bay the need for medication, injections and the numerous and terrible things that can and will happen to you if you just ignore it.

Would you like to know how many of you are *not* doing it right at the moment? According to the most recent study from the Institute of Health and Welfare only eighteen percent (that's less than two out of every ten) diagnosed diabetics have a co-ordinated chronic disease management plan. Diabetes is a chronic disease and you should speak with your GP about putting your plan in place. Ignoring this vital management of your condition is something my doctor calls "the great Australian *she'll be right mate* or *ostrich* syndrome".

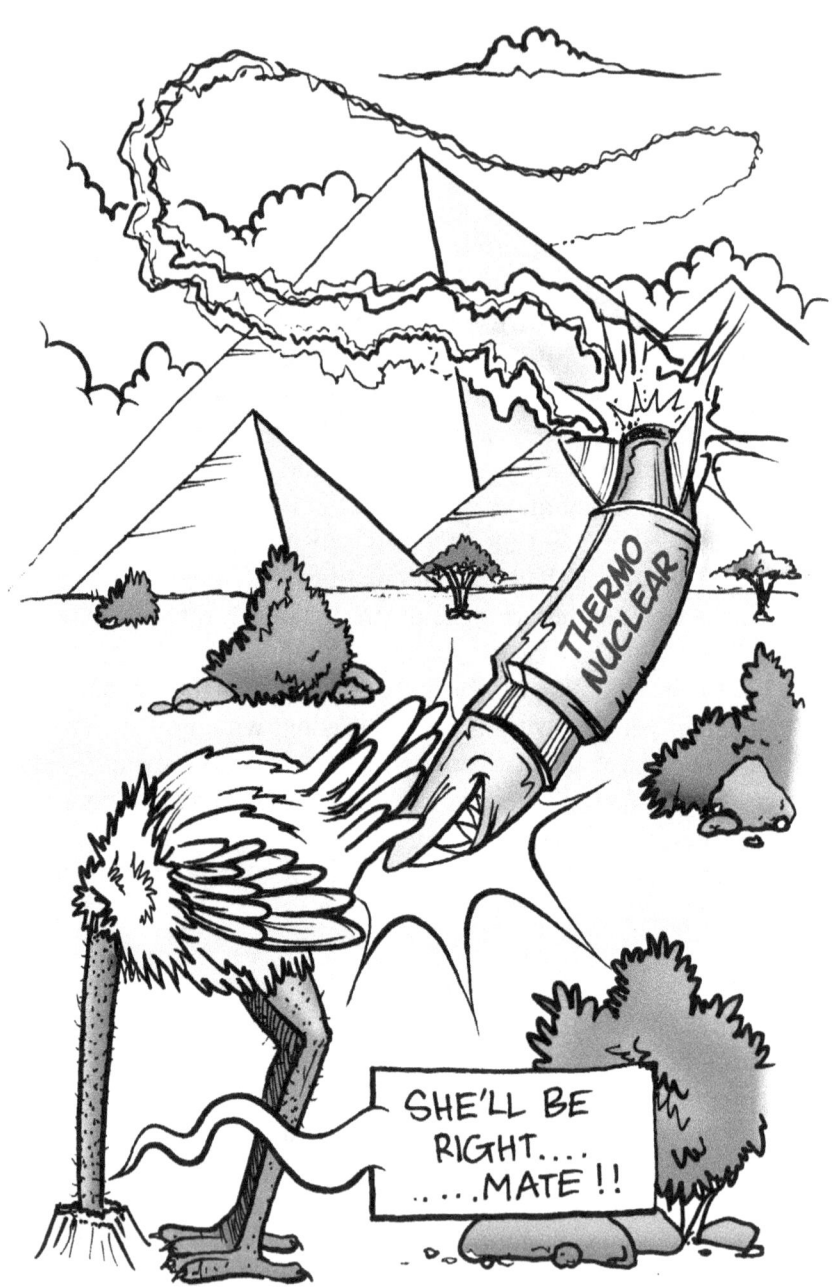

Control versus "cure"

I call the "ostrich syndrome" stupid and irresponsible – and I make no apologies for doing so. If you have been diagnosed with diabetes or pre-diabetes you simply cannot (and certainly should not) go on living your life without any adjustment for the fact that your body is nurturing a potentially life threatening, debilitating and painful chronic disease just because you're not exhibiting symptoms... yet.

The ostrich principle (otherwise known as the "she'll be right syndrome") is alive and well. For some the instrument has not been invented that can measure their indifference to their condition and they remind me a little of Winnie the Pooh when he said, "There's an alarming increase in the number of subjects of which I know nothing about!"

Let's just go back to Jason for a moment – remember he kept his condition under control with diet and exercise alone for nine years. Only after nine years did he graduate to a mere one tablet a day and he has the potential to retain this status for years to come. But here's the point about this story... no matter how good you are diabetes can *not* be cured. Once established it will persistently progress no matter how many people tell you otherwise, no matter how much you want to believe it isn't true, no matter how convincing the "30 day cures" available on the internet are – you are just kidding yourself. *Pre-diabetes* can be turned around... in *some* cases... but once you have it, you have it for life. Make it a long one.

Having said that, Gold Medal Olympians, movie stars, explorers, leaders of nations and senior executives all function very well and lead pain free and fulfilling lives with their diabetes – when they manage it properly.

Of course you can live on planet "who gives a ****" with a population of one and continue to demonstrate all the restraint of an average Roman orgy if you want to. It *is* your life and it *is* your choice.

Here's an interesting little piece of trivia for you. Once upon a time, in a land not so very far, far away, when a citizen went to have their driving license renewed they did not have to show medical evidence of their safe ability to drive if they were a Type Two diabetic on oral medication. Only insulin requiring diabetics needed to show medical evidence (the rationale of the esteemed and wise leaders of the nation being that only insulin requiring diabetics stood the risk of becoming a road hazard by suffering from a hypoglycaemic low if their diabetes was not correctly managed). However, a deep dark cloud of ignorance and denial had descended over the beautiful island nation and the Road Traffic Authority began to recognise that there were so many irresponsible diabetics on oral medication out there that, with great sadness and regret, they were forced to introduce the necessity for all diabetics on any level of medication to prove their medical stability before renewing their driving licenses - for fear of the safety of other good citizens on the road. Why is it so?

Surely only an insulin requiring diabetic is at risk of becoming a traffic hazard? *Not so*! It is now statistically recognised that there are so many irresponsible and uncontrolled Type Two diabetics on only oral medication that their cognitive abilities are too impaired to be considered safe drivers. Today anyone with an HbA1c reading over 9 (that's 75 in the US scale - the HbA1C is different from the daily glucose reading) requires a "conditional" license due to having glucose readings that are consistently *too high.* Consequently all medicated diabetics need to produce a doctor's certificate these days to have their driving license renewed. One doesn't need to jump to conclusions as a result of this change in policy… just take a tiny step and there conclusions are!

On top of eating right you must exercise, even if it's only a walk down the street or dancing at night, for at least thirty minutes a day. I either swim (when it's hot enough) or use the tread mill. I'm one of those multi-taskers who keeps the cell phone active while walking, or has someone sitting by the pool taking notes and/or making calls for me while I'm swimming – there's just no rest for the never weary! Multi-task or see it as relaxation – it doesn't matter how you do it, so long as you do it. Make no mistake – diabetes *is* a killer – in fact it is in the ***top ten leading causes of death*** in the Western World according to the Bureau of Statistics and here are a few other interesting numbers:

- 32% of all avoidable hospital admissions every year in Australia are due to diabetes! That is a staggering number!
- It costs the government up to twelve times as much to care for a diabetic with complications as it does to care for one who has been responsible and managed their condition to the best of their ability.
- Around 90% of all non-trauma limb amputations per year in Australia are due to diabetes.

Do you still think it's something you don't need to take seriously? To quote the Diabetes Australia website:

Q: Can Type Two diabetes be cured?
A: Currently there is no cure for Type Two diabetes, however the condition can be managed effectively. Researchers throughout the world are working on a cure.

The cure versus control issue is perhaps the most hotly contested and debated in the diabetic discussion. If you have diabetes and you lose weight your glucose tolerance *can* return to normal (in some cases) but you still need to maintain the lifestyle that brought the tolerance back to normal or the situation will revert back again. Some people see this as "cure" but technically it is not because otherwise you could progress with your life as someone without diabetes without the fear of your glucose tolerance slipping backwards and hence the risk of everything we have discussed. Once established diabetes will never "go away" and it can progress no matter what you do. It is only by careful and constant management and monitoring that you can significantly decrease your risk of adverse side effects progressing and (*in some cases*) even reverse your glucose tolerance to normal levels if you maintain your vigilance. Diabetes type two is many different diseases, not just one, so as I have said repeatedly in this book there is no "one size fits all" approach to managing it. The only one rule that does apply to everyone is you must have a chronic disease management program in place with your professionals on diabetes and you need to maintain your management every day... for life. This is the difference between control and cure. The wording of this paragraph has been approved by:

Professor Paul Zimmet

AO MD PhD FRACP FRCP FTSE

- **Director Emeritus & Director International Research Victor Smorgon Diabetes Centre, Baker IDI Heart and Diabetes Institute**
- **Foundation Director of the International Diabetes Institute**
- **Adjunct Professor, Harvest Alliance School for Indigenous Health, Monash University**

I understand why people want to believe they can just make this go away and I know there is a wealth of information and many so-called professionals and experts who will tell you that Type Two diabetes can be "reversed" or "cured". I am not an expert and you have no reason to listen to me – except that my information is coming from a lifetime's first-hand experience, a lifetime of mixing with some of the most brilliant medical minds in the world and information that has come directly from the national official body on this condition in this country – perhaps that will give me some credibility with you when I say that I don't care if your nurse, your best friend, or even your doctor has said that diabetes can be cured. Normal blood work without medication, after diabetes has been established, is *not* a reversal or cure – it is control. It trivialises a non-trivial chronic disease, it is irresponsible and inaccurate to say otherwise – and here's why it is irresponsible…

If you believe you are cured, as opposed to controlled, you are going to stop your tests, revert to old eating habits and stop exercising, thinking you have nothing to worry about. Do you know what will happen then? The disease, which is still there, lurking in the background, waiting to fire its torpedos at you, will think, "Beauty mate" and then…… *KA-POW*.

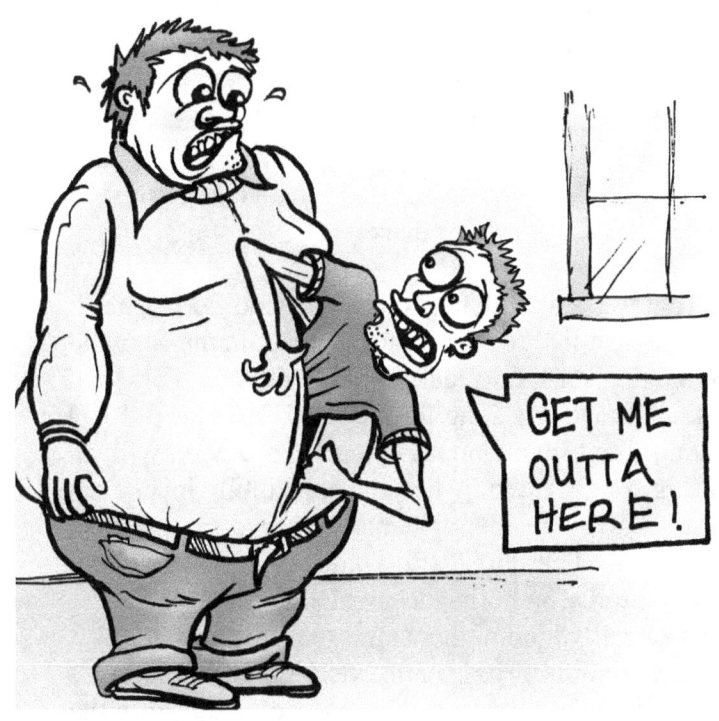

ABOUT THE FILM

In Australia we are actually doing well (in world terms). The place that Alby just about calls home these days, Micronesia, has the highest incidence of diabetes in the world and even in the USA 25% of the population are pre-diabetic (that's approximately *eighty million* people).

Too many people do not understand the risks and think of diabetes as a "lifestyle" disease which can be "cured". Just last week I heard of a case where a lady was hospitalised close to death with liver failure from having unknowingly had Type Two diabetes for two years with no symptoms.

21st April, 2012, the "**Alby Mangels – Adventure Bound**" series commenced airing on Channel One HD in the prime time Saturday night position. More than half of the seventy episodes have never been seen in Australia before but broke all ratings records when they aired in the US. Alby only agreed to come back to the forefront with his action-packed series for one reason – to give a voice to the important messages about diabetes.

Already my friend, the pop singing legend Leo Sayer, has agreed to be a live to camera test subject in the film and child singing sensation Jackie Evancho (New York) will be providing the theme song for the film. Ten year old Jackie Evancho shot to fame on *America's Got Talent* with an inspiring song written by her uncle, resulting in a personal invitation from President Obama for her to sing in the White House, February 2012. Diabetes is rife throughout Jackie's family, on both sides, which is why she is enthusiastically lending her support to this important project. In addition Herb Armstrong, grandson of the legendary Louie Armstrong, has agreed to appear in the film. Herb, a diabetic himself, sings with the voice of his famous grandfather and has the rights to Louie's songs, including the iconic and timeless "What a Wonderful World".

Alby will be meeting with world renowned specialists and personalities in bringing this vital message to the world, including prominent figures in the UK and France, an endocrinologist, a diabetic dietitian, a Professor on behavioural patterns that can lead to diabetes and others. He will be including visually spectacular settings on the world stage where diabetes is a major issue (such as Micronesia and Aboriginal Australia) and addressing many topics about the condition that most people living with the condition rarely consider.

In making a film for the global market we will also take into consideration that people in some countries do not have access to dietitians and educators who specialise in diabetes.

Alby says, "I feel I have a duty to use the celebrity fans have given me to make a positive difference in the world and this condition affects so many people, millions of whom don't even realise they have it, I consider it an honour to wake people up into getting tested. Who knows, perhaps the life this saves could be yours?"

Although Alby is neither a medical professional nor a psychologist, he has learned more about indigenous cultures, diets and health issues during his 40 years of travelling to some of the most remote regions of our planet than most people could imagine there is to know. The film script has been structured in such a way as to appeal to an audience that Diabetic Associations and Federations alone would not normally reach. Due to the professional nature of these bodies they are bound by certain codes of conduct and language, which is why this book could not be officially endorsed by them. While we understand and respect that position the fact is that the statistics prove most diabetics and pre-diabetics do not (and will not) read material that is dry, technical, complicated and overwhelming. While the official bodies are duty bound to present their information in a certain manner we are not so we can speak as real people to real people in a manner we hope they will really enjoy and hopefully benefit from.

While the tone and language I use is not endorsed every piece of information contained here has been verified.

It is our intention to speak to the governments of both Australia and America to encourage them to make this film available in every school in both Australia and US and roll it out globally thereafter.

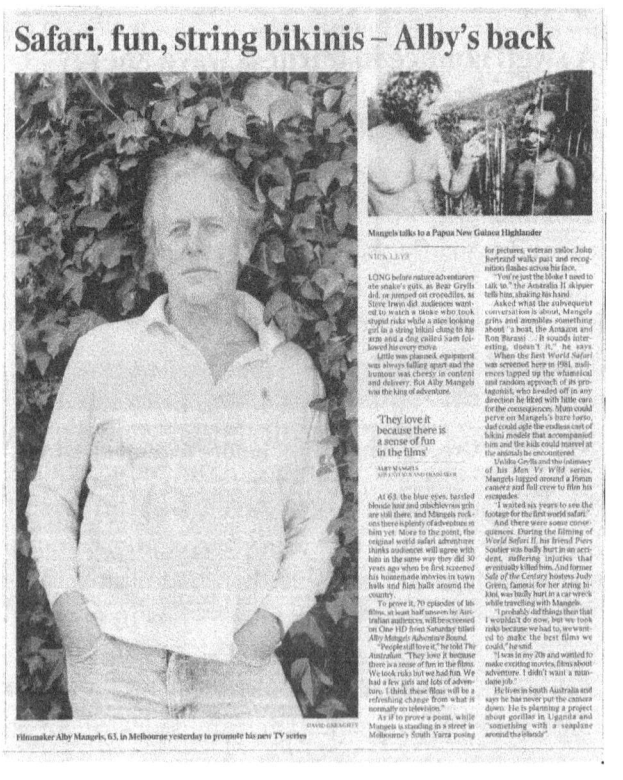

Recent media – page 3 – The Australian

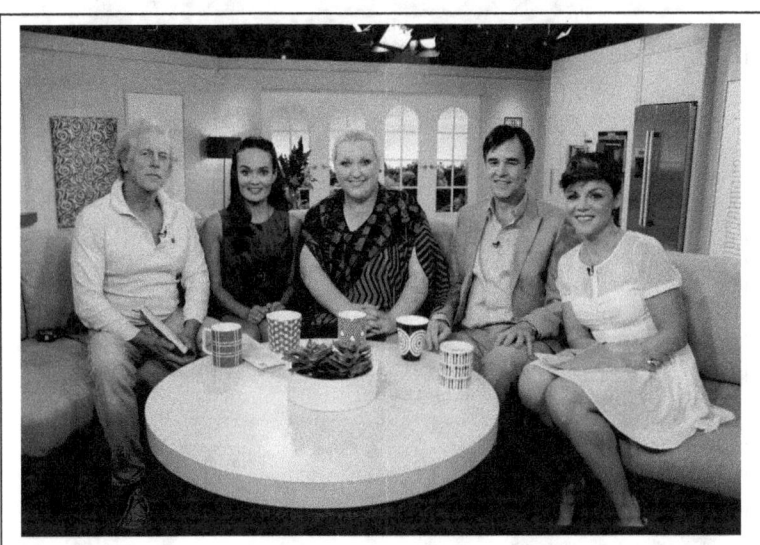

Alby on Channel Ten's "The Circle"
April 2012

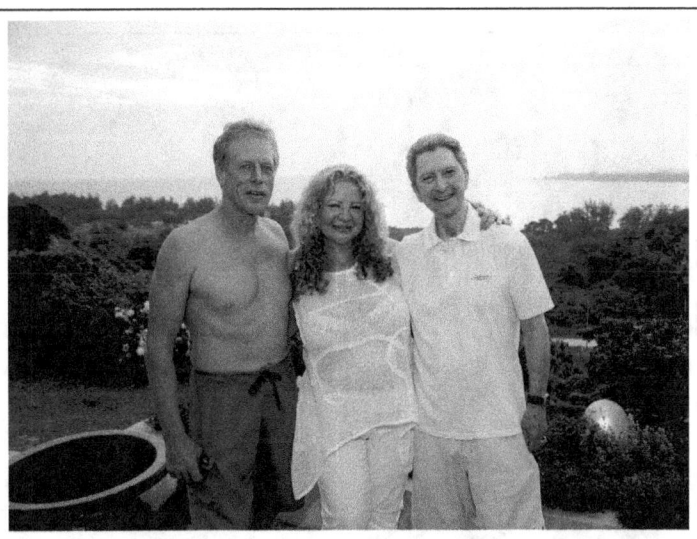

Alby, Lynn and veteran Hollywood producer Paul Mason (US script consultant and sales agent for the diabetes film) at Paul's holiday home in Port Vila

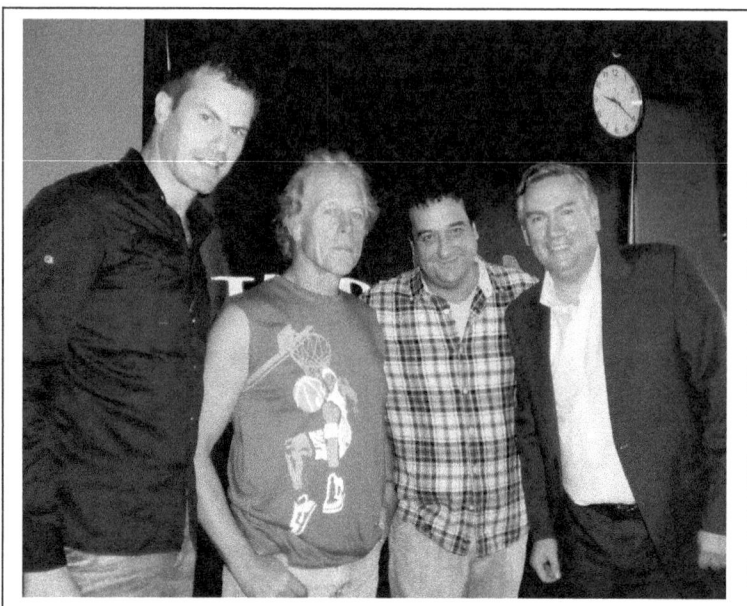

**Alby with Eddie McGuire & Co – Triple M radio
Melbourne interview – April 2012**

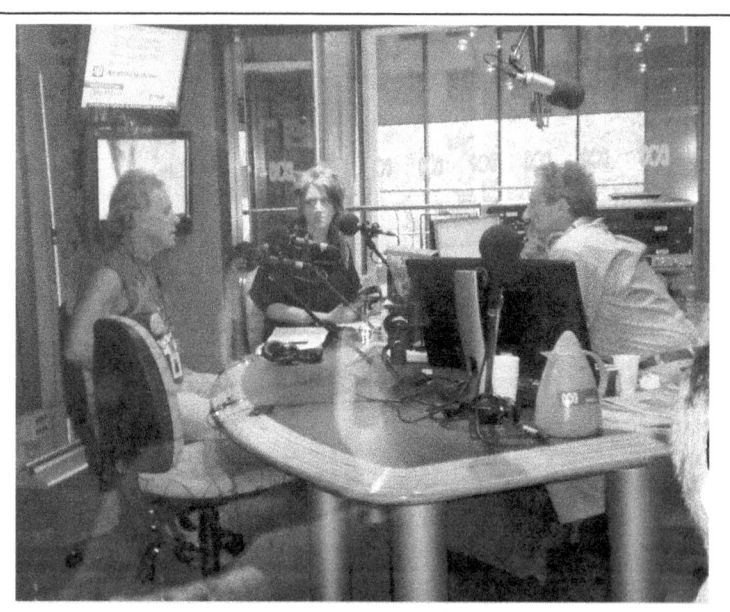

**The Conversation Hour – ABC radio Melbourne
April 2012**

METABOLIC SYNDROME

At the request of my doctor I am including some information here about Metabolic Syndrome. There aren't a lot of fluffy bunny rabbits in this chapter I'm afraid. Having read through the source information which follows (source: **betterhealth.vic.gov.au**) I understand why my doctor thought it was important for me to include and for everyone to read up on these details. There would be very few of us who are completely immune from one or more of the factors mentioned in this article, so while it's a bit dry – please read, digest, appreciate and then talk to your own doctor about it. It is important to understand because every one of the factors relating to Metabolic Syndrome link and interact with each other – monitoring and management is the most effective weapon in your arsenal to guard against the possible nasty ramifications, so please – read on.

Metabolic syndrome is a collection of disorders that occur together and increase your risk of developing Type Two diabetes or cardiovascular disease (stroke or heart disease). The causes of metabolic syndrome are complex and not well understood, but there is thought to be a genetic link. Being overweight or obese and physically inactive adds to your risk. Metabolic syndrome is sometimes called syndrome X or insulin-resistance syndrome.

As we get older, we tend to become less active and may gain excess weight. This weight is generally stored around the abdomen. This can lead to the body becoming resistant to the hormone insulin. This means that insulin in the body is less effective, especially in the muscles and liver.

More than twenty-five percent of Australian adults have metabolic syndrome. This is higher in people with diabetes.

A group of conditions that occur together

Metabolic syndrome is not a disease in itself, but a collection of risk factors that often occur together. A person is classed as having metabolic syndrome when they have any three or more of:

- Central (abdominal) obesity – excess fat in and around the stomach (abdomen)
- Raised blood pressure (hypertension)
- High blood triglycerides
- Low levels of high density lipoproteins (HDL) – the 'good' cholesterol
- Impaired fasting glucose (IFG) or diabetes. IFG occurs when blood glucose levels are higher than normal, but not high enough to be diagnosed as Type Two diabetes.

Insulin resistance

Insulin resistance means that your body does not use the hormone insulin as effectively as it should, especially in the muscles and liver. Normally, your digestive system breaks down carbohydrates into glucose, which then passes from your intestine into your bloodstream. As your blood glucose level rises, your pancreas secretes insulin into your bloodstream. Insulin allows glucose to move into your muscle cells from your blood. Once inside a cell, the glucose is 'burned' – along with oxygen – to produce energy.

When a person has insulin resistance, the pancreas needs to release more insulin than usual to maintain normal blood glucose levels. It is thought that more than a quarter of the population has some degree of resistance to insulin.

The link to diabetes

Insulin resistance increases your risk of developing Type Two diabetes and is found in most people with this type of diabetes. If the pancreas can't produce extra insulin to overcome your body's resistance, your blood glucose levels will rise and you will develop impaired fasting glucose, impaired glucose tolerance (IGT) or diabetes. People with Type Two diabetes frequently also have other features of metabolic syndrome and a significantly increased risk of cardiovascular (heart and blood vessel) disease.

Central obesity

Central obesity is when the main deposits of body fat are around the abdomen and the upper body. The greater your waist circumference, the higher your risk. A person's risk for central obesity varies depending on their gender and ethnic background.

As a general rule, if your waist measures 94 cm or more (men) or 80 cm or more (women), you probably need to lose some weight. Men from Middle Eastern, South Asian, Chinese, Asian-Indian, South and Central American ethnic backgrounds are considered at risk if their waist measures 90 cm or more.

High blood pressure (hypertension)

In the absence of other risk factors, hypertension occurs when a person has a blood pressure higher than 140/90mmHg. This may be due to genetics, lifestyle or other diseases such as kidney or cardiovascular disease. High blood pressure also increases your risk of developing cardiovascular disease, stroke and kidney disease.

The ideal blood pressure range is less than 130/80 mmHg (or lower, if other diseases are present), but everyone is different. Consult your doctor to find the right target for you and make sure your blood pressure is checked regularly.

Lifestyle changes such as regular physical activity, not smoking, reducing the amount of sodium (salt) in your diet, reducing stress, limiting alcohol and achieving a healthy body weight may help, but sometimes medication is required.

Cholesterol and triglycerides

Cholesterol is a fatty substance that we make in our liver. LDL (low density lipoproteins) cholesterol can block arteries by building up on the walls of blood vessels. HDL (high density lipoproteins) cholesterol helps protect against this build-up of fatty blockages.

Triglycerides may come from foods we eat, but they are also produced by the liver. Drinking excess alcohol can contribute to an increase in triglycerides. If you are insulin resistant, you are likely to have higher-than-normal triglyceride levels. High blood triglycerides tend to be associated with low levels of HDL cholesterol – the 'good' or protective cholesterol.

Raised triglycerides and reduced HDL cholesterol increase your risk for atherosclerosis (narrowing of the arteries), which is a contributing factor in heart disease. Excess weight or obesity is also a risk factor in itself for conditions such as high triglyceride levels, high blood pressure and atherosclerosis.

Impaired glucose tolerance (pre-diabetes)

Impaired fasting glucose and impaired glucose tolerance are sometimes referred to as 'pre-diabetes'. They occur when your blood glucose level is higher than normal, but not high enough to be called diabetes. People who have impaired glucose tolerance or impaired fasting glucose can develop diabetes unless lifestyle changes are made.

Does one condition trigger others?

All of these conditions are interlinked in complicated ways and it is difficult to work out the chain of events. Which condition – if any – is the main trigger? Some researchers consider that obesity could be the starting point for the metabolic syndrome.

Reducing your body weight and participating in regular physical activity may improve your triglyceride and cholesterol levels, lower your blood pressure and increase your body's response to insulin. This may help prevent you from developing Type Two diabetes and cardiovascular disease.

Ways to reduce your risk

More than half of all Australians have at least one of the metabolic syndrome conditions. Suggestions for reducing your risk include:

- **Incorporate as many positive lifestyle changes as you can** – eating a healthy diet, exercising regularly and losing weight will dramatically reduce your risk of diseases associated with metabolic syndrome, such as diabetes and heart disease.

- **Make dietary changes** – eat plenty of natural wholegrain foods, vegetables and fruit. To help with weight loss, reduce the amount of food you eat and limit foods high in fat or sugar. Reduce saturated fats, which are present in meat, full-cream dairy and many processed foods. Stop drinking alcohol or reduce your intake to less than two standard drinks a day.
- **Increase your physical activity level** – regular exercise can take many different forms according to what suits you best. Try and do at least 30 minutes of exercise on at least five days of each week. Also try to avoid spending prolonged periods of time sitting down, by standing up or going for a one-to-two minute walk.
- **Manage your weight** – increasing physical activity and improving eating habits will help you lose excess body fat and reduce your weight.
- **Quit smoking** – smoking increases your risk of cardiovascular disease, stroke, cancer and lung disease. Quitting will have many health benefits, especially if you have metabolic syndrome.
- **Medication may be required** – lifestyle changes are extremely important in the management of metabolic syndrome, but sometimes medication may be necessary to manage the different conditions. Some people will need to take antihypertensive tablets to control high blood pressure or lipid-lowering medications (or both) to keep cholesterol within the recommended limits. The most important thing is to reduce your risk of heart attack, diabetes and stroke.
- Consult your doctor to decide what the best management strategy is for you.

Where to get help

- Your doctor
- An Accredited Practising Dietitian, contact the Dietitians Association of Australia Tel. 1800 812 942
- Baker IDI Heart and Diabetes Institute Tel. (03) 8532 1111
- Diabetes Australia – Vic Tel. 1300 136 588
- Heart Foundation Tel. 1300 36 27 87
- Quit Line Tel. 13 7848 (13 QUIT)
- In other countries please Google the nearest office to you for these services.

Things to remember

- The metabolic syndrome is a collection of conditions that often occur together and increase your risk of diabetes, stroke and heart disease.
- Some of the components of metabolic syndrome include obesity, high blood pressure, high blood triglycerides, low levels of HDL cholesterol and insulin resistance.
- Healthy eating and increased physical activity are the keys to avoiding or overcoming problems related to metabolic syndrome.
- Consult your doctor about ways to manage metabolic syndrome.

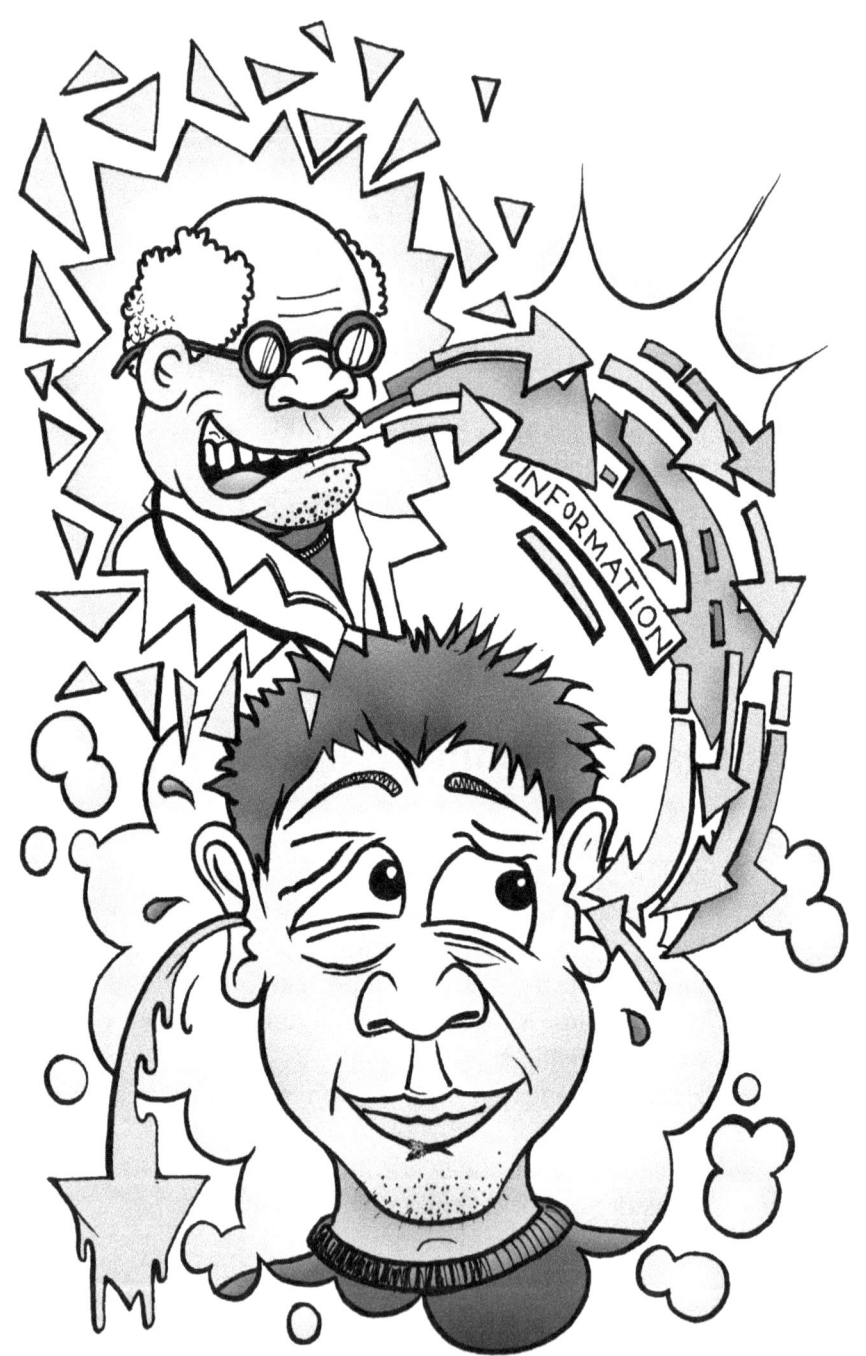

LATENT AUTOIMMUNE DIABETES OF ADULTS (LADA)

If you're not already completely confused – then this will definitely help. It will also explain why my doctor was so adamant that skinny people do **not** get Type Two diabetes.

To try and simplify this term, what it is essentially talking about is "slow onset Type One diabetes" being frequently misdiagnosed as the more common Type Two diabetes… which would explain why young, thin and active people are being diagnosed as Type Two diabetics when (perhaps) they are really slow onset Type One diabetics. Confused? Let me try and explain…

SOURCE: Wikipedia – paraphrased and abridged

Latent Autoimmune Diabetes of Adults (LADA) is also known as *Diabetes Type 1.5 (yes, you read right – Diabetes Type One AND A HALF).* The term was first coined in 1993 to describe "slow-onset Type One autoimmune diabetes in adults". I know this is all very technical, but please stay with me.

In Type One diabetes, the rate of beta-cell destruction is quite variable, being rapid in some individuals (mainly infants and children) and slow in others (mainly adults). The National Institute of Health defines LADA as "a condition in which Type One diabetes develops in adults." LADA is a genetically-linked, hereditary autoimmune disorder that results in the body mistaking the pancreas as foreign and responding by attacking and destroying the insulin-producing beta islet cells of the pancreas. Simply stated, autoimmune disorders, including LADA, are an "allergy to self."

Adults with LADA are frequently initially misdiagnosed as having Type Two diabetes. In a recent survey conducted by Australia's Type One Diabetes Network, one third of all Australians with Type One diabetes reported being initially misdiagnosed as having Type Two diabetes.

It is estimated that 20% of persons diagnosed as having non-obesity-related Type Two diabetes may actually have LADA (which still means that 80% of persons diagnosed as having non-obesity-related Type Two diabetes do not).

Not all people having LADA are thin or skinny, there are overweight individuals carrying LADA but not getting accurately diagnosed because of their weight. Moreover, it is now becoming evident that autoimmune diabetes may be highly under diagnosed in many individuals who have diabetes and that the body mass index levels may have rather limited use in connection with latent autoimmune diabetes. Also, many physicians or diabetes specialists don't recognize LADA, some may not even know the condition actually exists and so LADA is commonly misdiagnosed as or mistaken for Type Two diabetes.

If you think this might apply to you and your doctor hasn't discussed it with you yet, then bookmark this chapter and take it along to discuss with your physician (I expect to receive a lot of letters from physicians in the near future, but that's okay).

But wait! There's more. Even my own doctor hadn't heard about this one. Ready? Have you heard of "normal weight obesity"? It sounds like an oxymoron, doesn't it? Well, if your weight is normal or average, you may feel pretty good about your health. But according to a new Mayo Clinic study, you may look thin but really be too fat inside. You may have what is called normal weight obesity and if you do you are at risk of the same problems that are associated with being overweight or obese.

According to the new study, as many as thirty million Americans may mistakenly believe they are at a healthy weight but they really have an unhealthy percentage of body fat. Therefore, a woman whose weight is normal for her height and age but whose body fat is 30 percent or greater would be considered to have normal weight obesity. Among men of normal weight, body fat percentage should be less than 20 to 25 percent or else they are considered to be normal weight obese.

There's a You Tube you can watch on this subject here:
http://www.youtube.com/watch?v=H29a9P0YV38

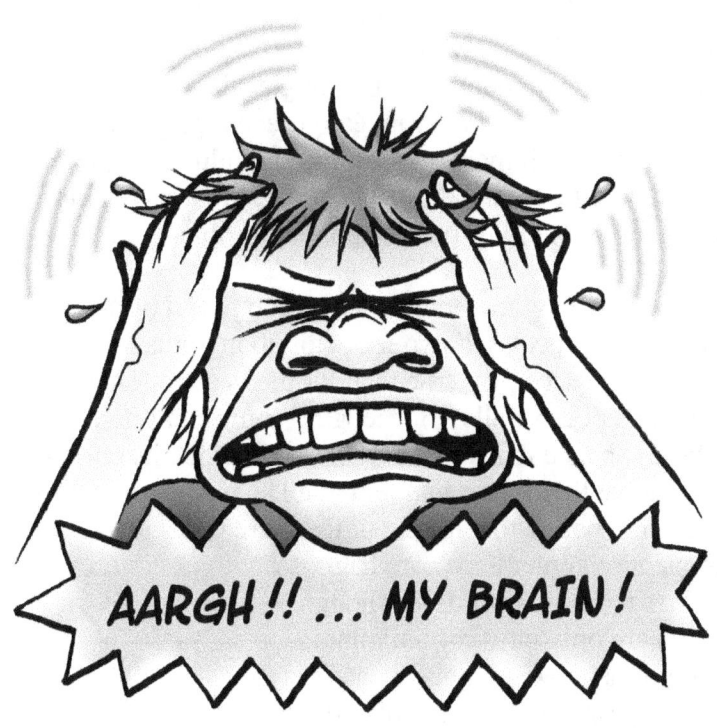

AARGH !! ... MY BRAIN !

PREVENTION IS BETTER THAN CURE – Talk to your doctor

This doesn't just apply to diabetes but rather to our general well-being. No matter what our state of health it is prudent to have an annual physical and check up but not everything shows up in a blood test. As an extreme example (given to me by my doctor) erectile dysfunction *can* be a result of lowered testosterone levels. You will appreciate my doctor wasn't talking about me as I don't suffer from either of those things! Seriously, though, the point he was making was that while erectile dysfunction and lowered testosterone levels may not seem life threatening conditions the lower testosterone levels *can* be as a result (for example) of sleep apnoea. There is a very nasty potential side effect of sleep apnoea and that is death! In fact another dear friend of mine, who was himself a medical doctor, did die from sleep apnoea. So all joking aside, a poor performance in the bedroom can be a symptom of something much more serious and shouldn't be ignored, nor should it be treated by only addressing the symptom and popping a pill to fix the apparent problem.

There is nothing too embarrassing, too trivial or too shocking to speak with your doctor about – that's what they're there for. It is true that our medical system in Australia doesn't allow for lengthy conversations with our GPs and hence many of us resort to naturopaths or other alternative therapists. I am not at all against naturopaths or other alternative therapists but there are times when only conventional medicine can diagnose and treat a condition. Even though Medicare only pays for ten minute appointments with your GP, at least once a year you should book a double or triple appointment to talk through everything that's going on in your life.

Doctors are not just prescription fillers. Prepare for your annual chat by writing down a list of things that are concerning you and questions you have. Any genuine and caring doctor will listen to you and you don't know what might alert him to a potential issue that has never occurred to you. My own doctor literally almost had me in tears when he explained how maybe one in one hundred patients ever really talk to him and how he could see that he could do so much more for them if they would only open up and then listen to his advice. A genuinely attentive medical practitioner cares about YOU. Sure there are doctors out there who only went to medical school because they wanted to own a Porsche and there are probably many who have become disillusioned, tired or cynical for various reasons but there are many, many doctors out there who actually care about improving and saving lives. If you don't have a conscientious and caring doctor like this then... change doctors. Your doctor should be your friend... for life.

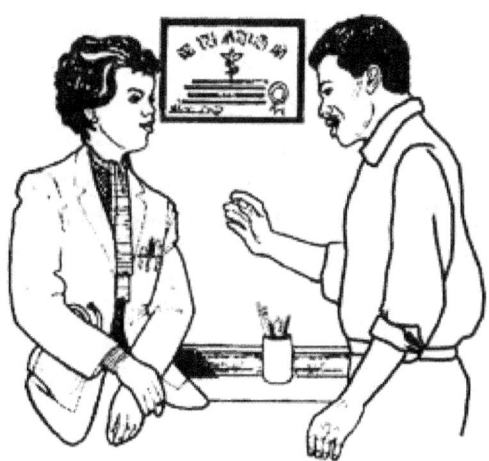

DIABETES IN PETS

Everything you do affects your glucose levels whether you have two legs or four.

Knowing whether your pet is showing symptoms of diabetes can save their lives.

What you should look for is:

- Weight loss, often despite increased appetite, although a lower appetite can also be a sign.

- If they are excessively thirsty or urinate more than usual.

- Pungent breath with a chemical smell.

- Or it could be they are slow to heal if they are injured.

Any of those things could be a sign of diabetes in your pet.

If you suspect your pet is diabetic take them to the vet immediately. Just like with humans, diabetes in animals needs to be closely managed for your pet to live a longer and healthier life. Just like with humans they will need a good diet, glucose monitoring and regular exercise.

Any vet can advise on the management of a pet with diabetes.

Show your animals that you love them as much as they love you and always be aware of their behaviour and appetite and please go and see a vet if you have any doubts at all.

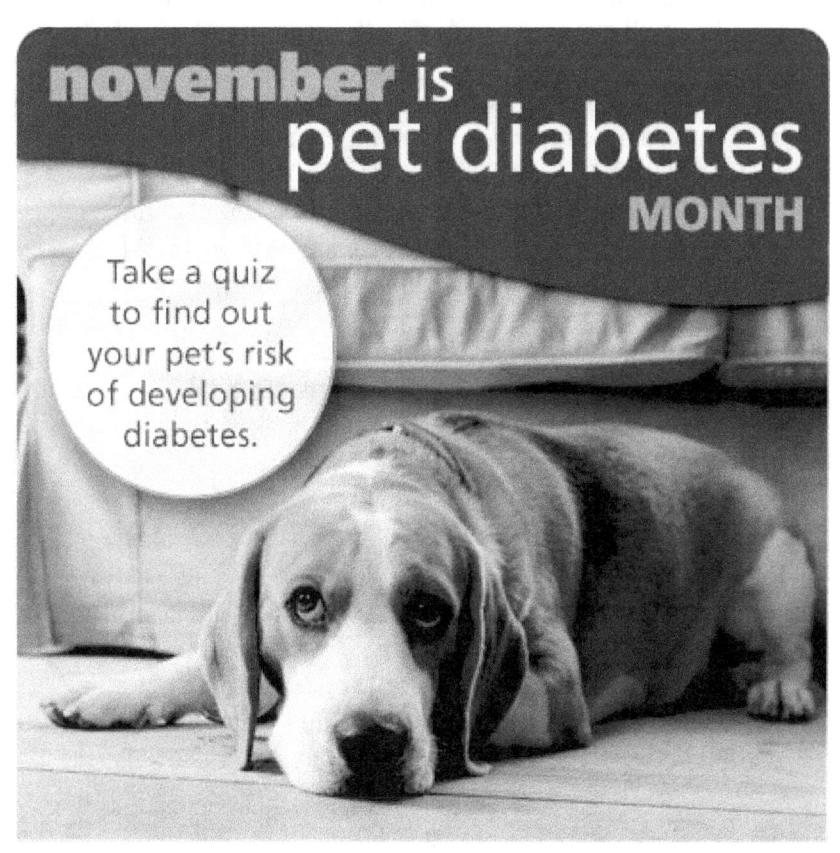

Go to this site:

http://www.petdiabetesmonth.com/survey-page.asp

MY PERSONAL STORY

To tell you where my personal story with diabetes began I need to back track a little. The reason for starting with this anecdote will become obvious as the story unfolds.

On the day my sister married her beau (and perhaps I could have picked a better time) I remember smiling at my brother-in-law to be and saying, "There's something I really need to tell you. You might be marrying the quieter more normal sister… but never lose sight of the fact that you'll be breeding from the same gene pool!"

The blood almost drained from his face! Nonetheless, the wedding proceeded and a while later they produced my first nephew, Lachlan. It was quickly apparent that their first child was definitely a product of the two of them – there was no need for concern about crazy Auntie Lynn's genes manifesting themselves. With that success under their belt they decided to try again. When I tell you that my last birthday card to my sister said on the outside "I'm smiling because you're my sister…" while on the inside it read "… and laughing my a*** off because there's nothing you can do about it" you will understand that when my second nephew started to display the latent traits of his crazy aunt – well, my sister and brother-in-law decided that this would be the end of baby making for them!

The second nephew, Joshua, and I have always been incredibly close. It's a bond, a friendship and an intuitive understanding that transcends my ability to put into words. Of course I am close to both my nephews – I adore them equally and would do anything for either of them – but there's just a synergy of spirit between Joshua and his crazy aunt. That said, here's what happened…

Day one – it was the week before Christmas (2011) and all through the house… no nothing was silent, it was more like a play about Faust!

The first sign I had that anything was wrong was a very mild, strange sensation in my leg. It was barely even noticeable, yet it waved a red flag to me. Most people wouldn't have noticed the symptom, but everything inside told me I knew what this was. Nonetheless, the holidays were almost upon us, my sister, brother-in-law and two nephews were about to arrive from Darwin, I was about to close a deal with Channel One to air Alby's entire "Adventure Bound" series of over seventy titles, I was finishing a riveting supernatural feature screenplay for a client in Sydney and as yet the most important detail hadn't been attended to – I hadn't stocked up the bar! Doctors could wait!!

Day two – 23rd December. Brisbane Airport is such a sedate and tranquil place two days before Christmas – NOT. With the stretch limo parked outside and mother all a twit of anticipation inside, we waited with anxious breath abated for the unbridled joy of throwing our arms around the family as they stepped off the long flight from Darwin. So we waited – and waited – and literally just as their plane touched down on the tarmac my mobile phone rang. It was the program manager from Channel One – and he wanted to talk deal! I didn't know what to be more excited about first! I frantically scribbled down the nuts and bolts of the deal and wondered if there was time to call Alby while my sister's plane taxied to the air bridge. After a brief and meaningful executive decision-making meeting with myself, I decided hang it all it was worth the risk. I rang Alby and was just finishing the call as my family emerged from their aircraft. Everything was wonderful. Who cared about Channel One anyway? Oh, wait a minute – I did! Then again the fact that my thirteen year old nephew's voice had just broken was rather diverting my attention.

My little boy was towering over me, he was speaking like a man and looking like one smoking hot young stud – even if he was still jail bate at that age. No really – who cared about Channel One?

Christmas day was just wonderful – well, it was "Santer's" time of year!

Boxing day was even more riotous. We had invited a few friends to eat left overs and have a drink at 2pm for an hour or so. It was 10pm before the last of the guests left and in between the first notable event was one of our recently insulin requiring diabetic neighbours suffering a hypoglycaemic low so severe we had to call an ambulance and he was hospitalised. Alby happened to phone from some far off land right in the middle of this chaos to say "Happy Holidays" and check on the progress of impending cyclone "Grinch" (as we'd named cyclone Grant) which was heading to my sister's home town of Darwin.

My sister, who had no idea about the fears I was harbouring, watched our neighbour being taken to hospital and said very quietly to me, "I thought all that was behind us" (meaning since my father's tragic passing over six years ago). I had to agree, but you can also imagine what was running through my mind. However, once we'd heard from the neighbour's wife that he was going to be okay, something seemed to snap in the rest of the guests and I think it was a serious case of **Carpe Diem** because the gathering turned into one of the most riotous events that has ever been hosted at "Santers on the Lake". Nonetheless, witnessing that low and knowing in my bones what was coming my way all weighed heavily on my mind.

Okay, I was guilty of having put on a few pounds (quite a few actually) and being inactive (as a writer it's an occupational hazard) I wasn't shy of a drink, I smoked and with my family history, well it was only a matter of time.

The image of my father's death still burned in my mind, as did the first occasion my father went down with a hypoglycaemic (hypo) low… and I do mean "went down". My mother and sister had been at the Melbourne Show with him. He said he was feeling hungry but it wasn't easy to find somewhere to get something to eat (he never went out without glucose on him after this). In only minutes he crashed to the floor in something that resembled an Epileptic fit. Only because of quick thinking nurses who happened to be looking after horses in fortuitously close proximity did a dreadful situation avert becoming a dire situation. And here we were all over again, the day after Christmas, thinking all that was behind us and my family having no idea whatsoever that I was fairly certain I had the condition myself. You can, I'm sure, imagine what was going through my mind.

Believing I was going to face a long and difficult illness, I emailed a resignation letter to Alby 27th December, 2011. Alby was understandably bemused – especially as I'd just landed the Channel One deal. And Alby wasn't the only one. My entire family thought I'd lost my marbles, moreover because Alby wasn't the one excited about the Channel One deal, I was. Of course none of them knew what was really going on inside my head. It seems crazy now but at the time it all made perfect sense to me.

Did I mention diabetes reacts adversely to stress?

28th December my elder nephew Lachlan flew to Melbourne and my sister and brother-in-law returned to Darwin, happy in the knowledge that cyclone Grinch had passed them by. This left only Joshua with mother and I through to New Year's Eve and the first week of January. During this time many phone calls took place… and not just between Alby and me.

Young Joshua was a babe magnet from when he was two years old in the playground. At age thirteen, as he was over Christmas, he had honed his skills quite considerably. I consider it to be only a matter of time before he gets RSI from texting his dozens of girlfriends into the wee hours of each morning. In one conversation with his mother/my sister I happened to say, "At this rate he's going to end up worse than Alby!" I didn't realise it but Joshua had overheard the conversation and wanted to know what I meant (especially given I'd just made a decision to part company with Alby and that was definitely not something Joshua wanted to replicate). I smiled and explained that Alby had once been tagged with a considerable reputation as a "ladies man". Joshua went away and thought about this and came back a few moments later with the following announcement…

"I am **not** going to be worse than Alby… I am going to be **better**!"

That's my boy!!!

Anyway, after many lengthy phone calls over several days between Alby and myself, during which time young Joshua assured me, "He's not going to let you go. I'm a man – and I know" we decided we wouldn't "divorce" after all, we would stay together for "the kids" (that's the range of Alby's films I manage for him). Joshua folded his arms, smiled broadly and simply said, "Told you so"!

Later I repeated the conversation about Joshua being worse than Alby… to Alby… adding in Joshua's punch line. I could almost see Alby grinning from a continent away, perhaps thinking, "Those are some big shoes to fill, son, good luck!"

So… my resignation only lasted a few days and on New Year's Eve we (Joshua, mother, friends and I) partied.

Saturday 7th January, 2012. My leg was beginning to drive me insane. Joshua was leaving the next day but I couldn't wait a moment longer. While he was still asleep (Joshua doesn't do mornings) I snuck out to my doctor, telling mom I had to run a few errands. I said nothing whatsoever to the doctor about diabetes, I didn't mention my family history – I wanted him to tell me it was nothing. Sure enough, however, diabetes was one of the first things he flagged. I was duly sent off for blood tests on Monday morning.

Sunday morning we waved a sad farewell to Joshua.

Sunday afternoon Andrew, the photographer who shot the Tanna job with Alby and I for New Idea, called asking if he could stay overnight the next day. If you could have seen our guest room! You would not believe how much carnage one thirteen year old boy can inflict on a single room. Of course we said yes to Andrew and promptly engaged industrial strength cleaning exercises in the spare room.

Did I mention diabetes reacts adversely to stress?

Monday 7am I stole away early for my blood test.

Monday 10am my clients from Melbourne arrived for their first day's brainstorming on my new book project.

Monday 4pm my clients departed for the day.

Monday 6pm Andrew arrived from Sydney for his sleep over.

Tuesday 7am Andrew departed.

Tuesday 10am my clients returned for the next brain storming session and mother was instructed I would take no calls.

Tuesday 11am a call was answered by mother from the doctor – recalling me from blood tests that mother had been unaware I had taken. Oh dear – that wasn't pretty!!!!!!!

Did I mention diabetes reacts adversely to stress?

Wednesday 8am I returned to the doctor. My fasting sugar readings were much higher than they should be and diabetes was suspected. My doctor started me on the lowest dose of oral medication, as even if diabetes wasn't confirmed something still needed to be done about the readings and he asked me to undertake the two hour, don't move, don't eat, don't breath, don't do anything you are not authorised to do, test to check my glucose tolerance and insulin absorption. Oh joy!

Wednesday 10am my clients returned.

Thursday 7am I underwent the glucose tolerance test.

Friday 10am I was recalled once again to the doctor – not a good sign. I made an appointment for the following week.

Saturday, even before the confirmed diagnosis, I went out and purchased a glucose meter and a form to register myself as a diabetic.

Monday 8am I returned to the doctor and the diagnosis was confirmed. My doctor spent ages and ages and ages with me explaining every little thing – he was so kind and concerned – but when he got to the part about telling me I could register as a diabetic and I pulled out the form and gave it to him along with the glucose readings I'd already been taking over the weekend, he was a little taken aback. "Right," he blinked. "I see… so you're on top of that one then!" At that point I explained my family history and lifetime of experience with the disease.

I was a little indignant that he said, "This is very exciting!"
Why should he make such an outrageous statement?
Because he was thrilled that I didn't go into shock or denial
as people normally do, I just went straight into, "Okay, this
is the situation, let's see how to deal with it." He was,
apparently, very excited and couldn't help repeating this
assertion several times. (I have since nicknamed him
"Doctor Excited" – although the first time he'll be aware of
this is when he reads this book.) Nonetheless he still
wanted more blood tests (I'll explain later).

At this point I told Alby, which might have explained to
him what had been otherwise inexplicable developments
over the holiday period. Within two days of that we were
planning to make a film together on diabetes. At that point
we both decided it was perfect timing for his "Adventure
Bound" series to be airing on TV as this gave us an
opportunity to speak with the media and raise awareness
about our planned diabetes project.

It was time to contact Diabetes Australia about the potential
Alby/Lynn co-production. With no contacts there
whatsoever I sent a cold email in through their website's
general form page. Twenty-four hours later the CEO
himself, Lewis Kaplan, made contact with me. Now *he* was
excited because he saw an Alby film as standing a better
chance of reaching more of the general public than
anything else ever could. So... that was good! I told Alby.
Then *he* got excited!! (I had to wonder how many men I
could make excited in one week?)

Then… guess what - I was recalled *again* from the latest
round of blood tests. This was beginning to become a royal
pain in the proverbial pyjamas and, dare I say, not a good
sign.

On return, yet again, to Doctor Excited, I learned my
cholesterol, while okay for a "healthy" person, was not

okay for someone with my condition. He spent forty minutes talking at me about this and that (in a scheduled ten minute appointment) and then complained, "You always do this to me. Now I'm behind time!" I HAD HARDLY OPENED MY MOUTH – HONESTLY!!!!!! Why was he so excited this time? The good news was that my triglycerides were normal and my HbA1c readings were not far into the diabetic range, which all proved I had (correction *we* had) caught my condition really early, which is outstandingly good news because most of the damage associated with diabetic complications has usually set in before the initial diagnosis takes place – hence why Lewis was so excited about a possible means of bringing this fact to people's attention.

Then came eye tests, foot treatments and my scheduled check ups with my dentist and gynaecologist – do you remember the gynaecologist from the introduction of this book?? Boy I was royally sick of seeing members of the medical fraternity by this point in time!

So, that's my story and as Doctor Excited said, I've turned a negative into a positive not just by losing weight and taking control of my own situation but in hopefully being able to help many others as well.

Now, please go to the mirror, look at yourself, and repeat this three times:

"If it is to be – it's up to me"

Thank you for sharing my journey with me.

Watch Channel One HD on Saturdays to see all of
Alby's "Adventure Bound" series, including
episodes never seen before in Australia
(and which broke all ratings records when they
aired in the US).

Visit these websites for more information:

www.LynnSanter.com

www.DontFeelLikeaPrick.com

www.SarisFilmProduction.com
(Requires Flash)

www.AlbyShop.com

www.TheMagicalScarecrows.com

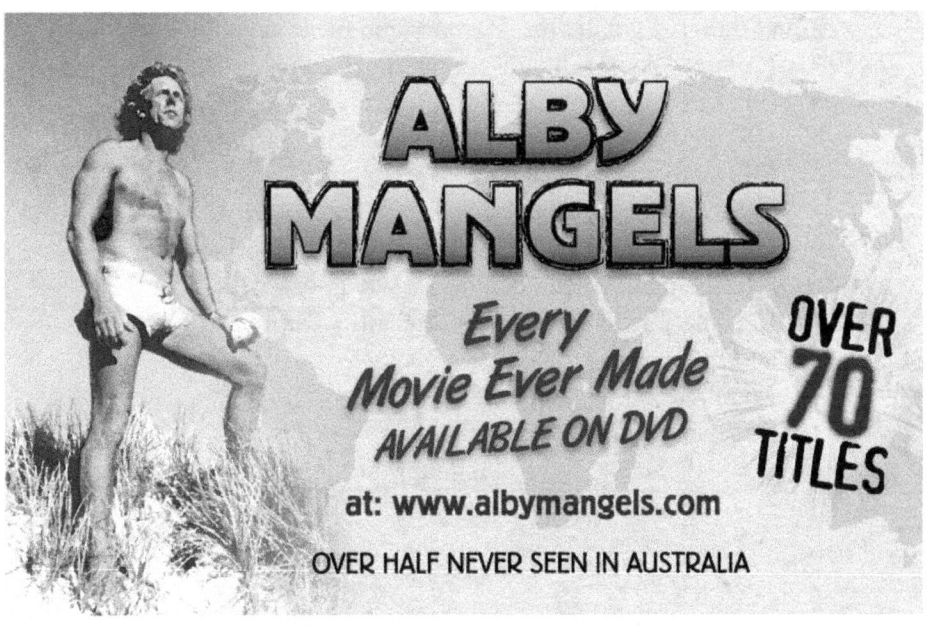

RESOURCES AVAILABLE TO YOU

The National Diabetes Services Scheme (NDSS) is an initiative of the Australian Government administered by Diabetes Australia. Through the administration of the NDSS, Diabetes Australia provides practical assistance, information and subsidised products to nearly 1,000,000 Australians diagnosed with diabetes. To register with the NDSS, applicants must be diagnosed with diabetes and hold or be eligible to hold a Medicare card and live in Australia. Sometimes visitors to Australia may be eligible through a Reciprocal Health Care Agreement with their home country. Subsidised products inc:

- Testing strips for checking blood glucose levels
- Free insulin syringes/pen-needles (if you require insulin)
- Subsidised insulin pump consumables (IPCs)
- Information services on managing life with diabetes.

Registration is free. Eligible persons can only be registered by their doctor or a Credentialed Diabetes Educator (CDE). For more information visit: **www.ndss.com.au**

Join Diabetes Australia. Membership benefits include:
- Preferred access and discounts for diabetes products and services
- Discounts on publications, travel, health insurance and footwear, amongst others
- Sales and advice on blood glucose meters
- Quarterly national and local magazines covering diabetes management, research and lifestyle issues
- Information and advice about healthy eating and physical activity
- Members-only web pages*
- Local community support groups*
- Some discounts from other suppliers*
  *only available in certain states

For costs in your state or territory call: **1300 136 588**

In other countries please Google the office nearest you.

EASY REFERENCE CHART

What follows is an easy reference chart to see if your daily readings indicate you have your condition well managed.

Diabetes Control Chart

	Excellent			Good		Poor					
HbA1c test Score	4.0	5.0	6.0	7.0	8.0	9.0	10.0	11.0	12.0	13.0	14.0
MEAN BLOOD mg/dL	50	80	115	150	180	215	250	280	315	350	380
GLUCOSE mmol/L	2.6	4.7	6.3	8.2	10.0	11.9	13.7	15.6	17.4	19.3	21.1

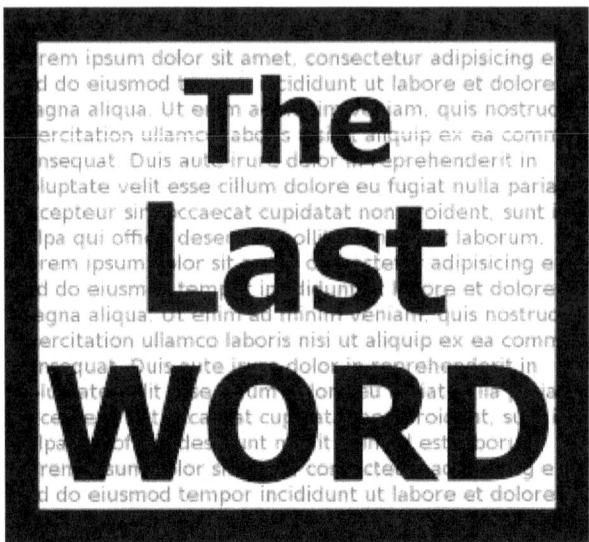

This idea of this book is to produce a consumable, fun, easy-to-read publication that is full of easy tips and tricks to help you manage your condition. In no way is this meant to replace the need for you to put a chronic disease management program in place and consult with professionals. My primary purpose is to encourage the two million Australians, eighty million Americans, seven million Britons and others who don't even know they have pre-diabetes and the 82% of diagnosed diabetics who do not have a chronic disease management program in place to see how vital it is that you do go and consult with the professionals.

While this book contains "verified" information diabetes is an extremely complicated and complex condition and even among the experts there is not always consensus on the "facts" (such as cure versus control and whether or not all type two diabetics will inevitably end up on insulin). I have taken every step within my power and accessed considerable resources to represent the expert views as they have been imparted to me and believe the content to be correct and accurate.